Political Economy, Health, and Aging

Little, Brown Series on Gerontology

Series Editors   Jon Hendricks
and
Robert Kastenbaum

W. Andrew Achenbaum
Shades of Gray:
Old Age,
American Values,
and Federal Policies
Since 1920

Linda M. Breytspraak
The Development
of Self in Later Life

Carroll L. Estes,
Lenore E. Gerard,
Jane Sprague Zones,
and James H. Swan
Political Economy,
Health, and Aging

Donald E. Gelfand
Aging: The Ethnic
Factor

Jennie Keith
Old People
As People: Social
and Cultural
Influences on
Aging and Old Age

Theodore H. Koff
Long-Term Care:
An Approach to
Serving the Frail
Elderly

Robert R. McCrae and
Paul T. Costa, Jr.
Emerging Lives,
Enduring Dispositions:
Personality in Adulthood

John Myles
Old Age in
the Welfare State:
The Political Economy
of Public Pensions

Jan D. Sinnott,
Charles S. Harris,
Marilyn R. Block,
Stephen Collesano,
and
Solomon G. Jacobson
Applied Research
in Aging: A Guide to
Methods and Resources

Martha Storandt
Counseling and
Therapy with
Older Adults

Albert J. E. Wilson III
Social Services
for Older Persons

Political Economy, Health, and Aging

Carroll L. Estes
Lenore E. Gerard
Jane Sprague Zones
James H. Swan

Aging Health Policy Center
University of California, San Francisco

Little, Brown and Company
Boston   Toronto

Library of Congress Cataloging in Publication Data
Main entry under title:

Political economy, health, and aging.

  1. Aged—Medical care. 2. Aged—Government policy.
3. Aged—Medical care—United States. 4. Aged—Govern-
ment policy—United States. 5. Aged—United States.
I. Estes, Carroll Lynn, 1938–
RA564.8.P65   1984   362.1'9897'00973   84–942
ISBN 0-316-25062-7
ISBN 0-316-25061-9 (pbk.)

Library of Congress Catalog Card Number 84-942

ISBN 0-316-25062-7

ISBN 0-316-25061-9 {pbk.}

9 8 7 6 5 4 3 2 1

ALP

Published simultaneously in Canada
by Little, Brown & Company (Canada) Limited

Printed in the United States of America

To
Philip R. Lee
whose insights and
commitment to social justice
inspired this work

Foreword

Where is it? In each of the billions of cells in our bodies? Or in our minds? Then, again, perhaps it is something that happens *between* people. Ought we not also take a look at the marketplace as well? And at the values expressed through our cultural institutions? Undoubtedly, the answer lies in all these factors—and more. The phenomenon of aging takes place within our bodies, in our minds, between ourselves and others, and in culturally defined patterns.

The study and analysis of aging—a burgeoning field—is deserving of an integrated spectrum approach. Now, Little, Brown and Company offers such a perspective, one designed to respond to the diversity and complexity of the subject matter and to individualized instructional needs. The Little, Brown Series on Gerontology provides a series of succinct and readable books that encompass a wide variety of topics and concerns. Each volume, written by a highly qualified gerontologist, will provide a degree of precision and specificity not available in a general text whose coverage, expertise, and interest level cannot help but be uneven. While the scope of the gerontology series is indeed broad, individual volumes provide accurate, up-to-date presentations unmatched in the literature of gerontology.

The Little, Brown Series on Gerontology:

—provides a comprehensive overview
—explores emerging challenges and extends the frontiers of knowledge
—is organically interrelated via cross-cutting themes
—consists of individual volumes prepared by the most qualified experts

—offers maximum flexibility as teaching material

—ensures manageable length without sacrificing concepts, facts, methods, or issues

With the Little, Brown Series on Gerontology now becoming available, instructors can select the texts most desirable for their individual courses. Practitioners and other professionals will also find the foundations necessary to remain abreast of their own particular areas. No doubt, students too will respond to the knowledge and enthusiasm of gerontologists writing about only those topics they know and care most about.

Little, Brown and Company and the editors are pleased to provide a series that not only looks at conceptual and theoretical questions but squarely addresses the most critical and applied concerns of the 1980s. Knowledge without action is unacceptable. The reverse is no better.

As the list of volumes makes clear, some books focus primarily on research and theoretical concerns, others on the applied; by this two-sided approach they draw upon the most significant and dependable thinking available. It is hoped that they will serve as a wellspring for developments in years to come.

Acknowledgments

This book is the product of a genuinely collaborative effort, not only among the authors, but with many of our colleagues and companions as well. To start, we thank Jon Hendricks, one of the editors of this series, for his urging us to write the book in the first place, for his careful reading and rereading of the manuscript, and for his invaluable suggestions.

Among those who have had special intellectual influence on our work as sociologists are Robert Alford, Herbert Blumer, Randall Collins, Alvin Gouldner, Joseph R. Gusfield, Howard E. Freeman, and Edmund H. Volkart. The writings of Manuel Castells, James O'Connor, John Walton, and Eric Olin Wright have been key to our thinking in political economy. We are particularly indebted to Philip R. Lee, whose understanding of the complex territory, politics, challenges, and nuances of health policy aided us in every phase of this book. Equally important has been the colleagueship and friendship of Maggie Kuhn, founder and National Convener of the Gray Panthers, who strengthened our determined commitment to exploring the linkages among health, capitalism, class, and age. Mary Lee Ingbar fostered professional growth in her teaching of health economics.

We are deeply grateful to our families, informal, legal, and extended, for the many types of support they ceaselessly offered. Husband Philip Lee and daughter Duskie Lynn Gelfand rendered invaluable emotional support and sacrificed time that would have been spent with Carroll Estes, making her work on this book possible. Carroll Cox Estes, an author and feminist in her own right, gave her daughter the courage to write what she believed. Yolanda Anaya assisted in multiple ways with household support. For Lenore Gerard,

Ellen Gerard first sparked her granddaughter's compassion for and investigation into the social experience of old age; Leonora Avery grounded her daughter's theory in practical understanding of the nurse's role in long-term care and provided inspiration by her political acumen and moral commitments; Jak Dyer provided constant loving support. Paula and Charles Burr educated Jane Sprague Zones in all ways about living vitally at every age; Stacey Zones, Milo Sprague, and Isaac Zones take pride in rather than tolerate her work. Sandra Swan donated encouragement and tolerance of Jim Swan's long hours.

Our co-workers in the School of Nursing, the Aging Health Policy Center, and the Department of Social and Behavioral Sciences at the University of California, San Francisco, supported us in many ways. Ida VSW Red provided her exceptionally precise editorial talents. Norton Twite and our irreplaceable crew of wordsmiths, Sue Churka-Hyde and Emilie Cruger, brought us through the breach once again. We are grateful to all who endured the bumping of their work to send our new editions through the queue. Kerry McDermott and Francoise Case humored us by taking care of all matters great and small while our attention was turned to finishing this work. Elaine Benson, Robert Newcomer, Nancy Nienhuis, and Margaret O'Neill assured the continued smooth functioning of the Department and the Center.

Virginia Olesen's constant encouragement was especially important. Finally, we are indebted to Steve Wallace and the multiple generations of graduate students in the Seminar on Medical Sociology who have considerably sharpened our perspective on the topics of this volume. None of our associates, many of whom must remain unnamed, are responsible for the analysis and commentary that follow. We thank them all for their support.

Contents

Political Economy, Health, and Aging

Chapter

1

An Introduction to the Political Economy of Health and Aging

An analysis of health and aging from a political economy perspective emphasizes the broad implications of economic life for the aged and for society's treatment of the aged and their health. A political economy analysis also examines the circumstances for different classes and subgroups of older persons. It is a systemic view based on the assumption that old age cannot be understood in isolation from other problems or issues raised by the larger social order.

An analysis of the relationship of economic and social factors to the definition and treatment of health and old age requires an interdisciplinary and historical approach. Sociology, economics, and political science, as well as gerontology, epidemiology, and health services and health policy research, are relevant fields that contribute to a comprehensive framework. The political economy perspective calls theoretical and empirical attention to the socioeconomic determinants of health and illness in old age and to the policy interventions reflecting society's view of the elderly in the context of a capitalist economy. The lives of the elderly can be understood only in relation to the lives of other generations and segments of society, and in relation to the broader social and symbolic order. A political economy perspective examines

> the interrelationships between the polity, economy, and society, or more specifically, the reciprocal influences among government . . . the economy, social classes, strata, and status groups. The central problem of the political economy perspective is the manner in which the economy and polity interact in a relationship of reciprocal causation, affecting the distribution of social goods. (Walton, 1979, p. 9)

Recent work in the emerging field of the political economy of aging has attempted to show how the meaning and experience of old age and the distribution of resources are influenced by broad economic and political factors (A. Walker, 1980; 1981; Townsend, 1981; Estes, Swan, and Gerard, 1982; Olson, 1982; Myles, 1984; Nelson, 1983; Guillemard, 1982). This work has led to an increased awareness that public policy for the aged in general and health policy in particular mirror the structural arrangements of U.S. society and the distribution of political, material (economic), and ideal (values and beliefs) resources within it. In other words, public policy reflects and reinforces the "life chances" associated with each person's social location within the class, status, and power structures that comprise society (Weber, 1946). The lives of each succeeding generation are similarly shaped by public policy and the extent to which that policy is designed to maintain or to redistribute those life chances.

The problems of the aged and the policies and processes for treating them reflect the system of social and power relationships. The political economy analysis of health and aging therefore calls attention to: the sociopolitical context in which society views older persons and how this affects the elderly; the sociopolitical and economic causation of illness; the political and economic basis of health policies; the distribution of benefits that affect health; and the relative power of the professions, medical industries, corporations, and banks in framing the life chances of different subgroups of older persons. Thus one challenge is to understand not only how people interpret their private troubles (for example, health in old age), but also how these private troubles intersect with history and become public issues generating major societal responses through public policies such as Medicare (Mills, 1956). For example, historically, which social-structural features manifest change and elevate concepts of private troubles to the level of public issues? How do these public issues reflect the dominance and structural location of certain interests, institutions, and classes? How are the health and subjective experiences of individuals in old age shaped by these social forces? The structure and operation of the major societal institutions (for example, the family, the work place, the medical and welfare institutions) are of particular interest as they shape both the subjective experience and objective condition of the individual's aging.

The political economy perspective emphasizes

1. the social determinants of health and illness;
2. the social creation of dependency and the management of that dependency status through public policy and health services;
3. medical care as an ideology and as an industry in the control and management of the aging;

4. the consequences of public policies for the elderly as a group and as individuals;
5. the role and functions of the state vis-à-vis aging and health; and
6. the social construction of reality about old age and health that both undergirds and reinforces the institutional arrangements and public policies concerning health and aging in the society.

The social basis and etiology of health and illness is an analysis of the effects of poverty, stress, living conditions, nutrition, and work on patterns of death and disease. As Conrad and Kern (1981, p. 32) have indicated, "one of the most striking features about the distribution of disease is its relationship to poverty. By and large, death and disease vary *inversely* with social class . . . the poorer the population the more sick people and the higher the death rates." A broad conceptualization is required in order to account for the social origins of morbidity and mortality differences across different social classes and racial and ethnic groups (Conrad and Kern, 1981; Doyal, 1979).

Doyal's analysis (1979) goes further in tracing the origins of disease and illness to a nation's economic base of production. Although the unprecedented development of productive forces in capitalist nations has improved the standard of living for the population as a whole, "new hazards to health have been created . . . by the large-scale economic, social and technological changes which were a necessary part of this development" (Doyal, 1979, p. 47). Commodity production affects health in very important ways, such as in the areas of work-related disease and disability, environmental health hazards, and harmful commodities consumed by the general public. McKinlay's analysis (1981) of the political economy of illness focuses on the relationship between big business and patterns of disease. "Manufacturers of illness" are those "individuals, interest groups, and organizations which, in addition to producing material goods and services, also produce as an inevitable by-product, widespread morbidity and mortality" (McKinlay, 1981, p. 614). The food, tobacco, and pharmaceutical industries are an example. Thus, the social production of illness refers to the origins of ill health as a result of the production and consumption of commodities in advanced capitalist nations.

Medical care operates as a system of social relations. The different ways in which health and illness are defined and treated reflect the structural arrangements and resource disparities in the society.

Diagnosis and prescribed treatment must be seen in terms of power relations. Those who control the definitions of sickness and health also control access to medical care, the personal and public costs of that care in terms of the types of services reimbursed, and even the structure of the health care organization. Currently, both public money and professional effort are disproportionately expended on institutional (hospital and nursing home) services for the elderly. This reflects a definition of health and health care that is both a product of the professional dominance of medicine and a guarantee of a profitable industry.

While elaborating the macrosociological perspectives associated with a political economy approach, we must also consider the microsociological level. Particularly important are the theories of symbolic interaction, labeling, and deviance (Becker, 1963; Matza, 1969; Conrad and Schneider, 1980). These theories describe the social perceptions, processing, and treatment of individuals as members of a collective group in society. For example, the experience of growing old is "produced" socially in that it is "neither immutable nor 'given' by the character of external reality" of old age itself (Gusfield, 1975, p. 286).

How old age is regarded by members of the society is socially constructed by what is attributed or imputed to aging. These attributions, in turn, determine how old age is processed and treated by society. Thus the conceptualization of old age and of the aged as inherently sick or healthy is socially created in the sense that it is not determined solely by objective facts. It is the interpretation and ordering of perceptions of "facts" into ways of thinking and the relative power and influence of those who interpret and disseminate facts that create such conceptualizations (Gouldner, 1970). In this sense, the elderly do not have any problems other than those that experts, policy makers and the public media define as real for them (Estes, 1979). Such attributions are framed by available theories, methodologies, and research data that channel the conceptualization, conduct, analysis, and interpretation of data, as well as by the dominant social, economic, and political forces and intellectual fashions of the period (Gouldner, 1970).

A society's defining or labeling of old age has multiple levels of significance (Schur, 1971; Conrad and Schneider, 1980). First, it affects interpersonal relations (Becker, 1963; Thomas, 1970), as the literature on the looking-glass self and the self-fulfilling prophecy has amply demonstrated. What others think of us is a strong influence on what we think of ourselves (Scott, 1970; Rodin and Langer, 1980). Second, social labels both affect and reflect "collective rulemaking" (Conrad and Schneider, 1980), including the legal status of the elderly and the public policies that are formed to deal with elders and their health. Third, both the social relations and rule making influence how the elderly are "processed"—that is, how they are treated by public policy and societal institutions.

A common practice in our society is to equate aging with traditional notions of illness (that is, a pathological or abnormal condition). Associated with this propensity to think of old age biologically is the tendency to link aging with disease. The linking of aging to illness expresses a negative judgment. As Conrad and Schneider have argued, "entities labeled an illness or disease [are] undesirable" (1980, p. 31). Thus there are consequences independent of the effects of the biological condition of the organism, for "a social state is [then] added to a biophysical state" (Friedson, 1970a, p. 223). Medical diagnosis influences behavior and shapes both the attitudes people hold toward themselves and the attitudes others take toward them (Conrad and Schneider, 1980).

Much labeling of the aged involves a focus on physical debility and physiological decline. Elders, "even in the absence of medically diagnosed pathology, are now expected to adopt a social role which has all the characteristics of a sick role" (Arluke and Peterson, 1981). Sick role expectations (first described by Parsons in 1951) applied to old people include withdrawal from the social world, reduction of normal social and occupational responsibilities, and becoming dependent on others in an imbalanced power relationship (Arluke and Peterson, 1981). The myth of pervasive debility in old age persists and can serve as a self-fulfilling function with regard to the loss of effectiveness and personal control (Rodin and Langer, 1980). Insinuations of loss of competence or mental illness are two major vehicles for ushering the elderly into protective custody or institutions for long-term care, in which the aged are particularly susceptible to external management. The medical profession, by attributing physical decline and consequent personal incompetence to the aging process per se, effectively "depoliticizes" (Zola, 1977) issues related to institutionalization or legal responsibility. Consequently, attention is focused on the individual and individual treatment, rather than on the social situation creating the problem. Yet human beings do not relinquish power over their lives without strong objection. Protestations by the elderly about their social situation and treatment are generally considered unseemly, leading to the application of age-stereotyped epithets such as "cantankerous," "crotchety," "dyspeptic," and so on.

Conrad and Schneider (1980) hypothesize that such "misbehavior" and the deviant labels attached to it are more likely to fall under the purview of medicine when the problem becomes a middle-class one rather than solely a lower-class one. Likewise, they posit that the probability of the medicalization of a social problem increases when there is a potential for economic profitability and previous systems of social control have failed. The overuse of prescription drugs exemplifies a commonly employed—and lucrative—means of controlling the behavior of those elders who are regarded as disruptive or deviant. The elderly are the most likely of all age groups to have drug-induced illness. Many of the drugs prescribed to institutionalized elders are tranquilizers, sedatives, and hypnotics. In addition, millions of noninstitutionalized elderly have "bought into" (that is, accepted) such drugs as a way of coping with stressful conditions (Lee and Lipton, 1982). The effect of tranquilizers, sedatives, and hypnotics is to diminish autonomy by reducing one's ability to engage in social interaction.

Statistics belie the notion that all, or even most, elders are sick and getting sicker. More older people in our society are living to advanced ages and prolonging their "productive" (that is, disease-free) life span (see Chapter 5). Nevertheless, the potential for acute and chronic health problems in old age remains. Many elders eventually face periods of decline and dependency. If, however, elders were permitted to enter times of illness without shame and guilt about dependency for personal care and financial support, and if health care and aging policies accommodated the social and economic needs of elders, old age would not be the burden it has become.

The Gerontological Focus

Society's limited understanding of health in old age (and thus of the most appropriate health policy interventions) may be explained in the context of the major theoretical perspectives that have dominated gerontological research and training in the United States. At least eleven theoretical themes in gerontology have been identified (John, 1982), no one of which, in itself, is adequate to explain the experience and process of aging. The field of gerontology also lacks a unifying conceptual framework to weave these themes into a comprehensive theory (Hendricks and Hendricks, 1981). Major fields of study with an influence on gerontology are biology and medical science, social psychology, sociology, and, more recently, epidemiology.

Biological Theories

First and foremost has been the dominance of biological theories of aging. These theories are concerned with physiological and anatomical changes in different organ systems of the body that accompany chronological aging. Also of interest are changes in molecular and cellular structures, immune systems, and hormones and enzymes, among others. Such theories seek to "explain the progressive loss of biological integrity over life" (Hendricks and Hendricks, 1981, p. 92). They are currently measured across four parameters—biochemical, anatomical, physiological, and behavioral

(Wallace, 1977). The wear-and-tear theory (parts of the human organism wear out as finite stored energy is used up) was one of the earliest ideas advanced by biologists but is now regarded with disfavor. Related to this is another widely accepted causal explanation of aging—the stress theory—which refers only to physical wear and tear from sudden and unexpected stressors over which one has no control (excluding sociopsychological strain) (Hendricks and Hendricks, 1981). More recent biological theories of aging are

1. genetic theory (a failure in DNA replication, transcription, or translation, or a malfunction in RNA or related enzymes);
2. autoimmunity theory (forbidden clones or similar mechanisms are capable of a minor attack on a variety of tissues, such attacks occurring with greater frequency with aging);
3. free radical theory (an increase in unstable free radicals produces deleterious changes in biological systems, for example, chromosome changes, accumulations of pigments, and alterations in macromolecules such as collagen); and
4. the theory that RNA tumor virus may play a role in the aging process.

Overall, medical science research is seeking to unlock the mysterious process of aging, the causes of morbidity and mortality, and the relationship between age and functional capacity. Also, observations in medical science research often are made independently of the insights of other research showing that "longevity is a consequence of the reciprocal influences of normal physiological aging and a wide range of social and environmental factors" (Hendricks and Hendricks, 1981, p. 91). The policy interventions suggested by research reflecting this narrow focus on biological processes produce contradictions. On the one hand, some fear the physical consequences of extended life spans (that is, more worn-out individuals extracting a high cost from society to support their medical and social needs) (Wallace, 1977). Others view increased longevity as an opportunity to expand productive human potential (Fries and Crapo, 1981) (see Chapter 5).

Social and Psychological Theories

Social and psychological theories of aging include disengagement, activity, personality, age-stratification, and socioenvironmental theories.

Disengagement Theory. Disengagement theory represents a structural-functionalist view of aging. The theory postulates that there is a mutual withdrawal between the individual and society, called "dis-engagement." Cumming and Henry (1961) describe this process as inevitable, intrinsic, unilateral, universal, and beneficial for both society and the aging individual. They argue that disengagement functions to prepare society for the requisite replacement of its members when they die and, at the same time, to assist the individual in preparing for death. The societal aspect of this theory (how "society" withdraws from the aged as an inherent, requisite functional process) has not been empirically studied. It has been assumed to exist on the basis of mandatory retirement, age discrimination, and other governmental policies that encourage disengagement by restricting certain types of involvement of older persons in the society.

Activity Theory. In contrast to disengagement theory, activity theory indicates that high activity results in high morale and high life satisfaction (Havighurst and Albrecht, 1953). Activity is essential to successful aging, as is the maintenance of the activity patterns of one's middle age. Lost social roles must be replaced by substitute roles and activities. The theory implies that to be adjusted, older people must extend middle-age patterns as long as possible. As an essentially classless and universal prescription for continued activity in old age, activity theory lends support to policies that assist in the social integration of the aged. Suggested policies would focus on recreational and social activities, as well as on a health orientation that assists the elderly in remaining active and socially integrated. For activity theorists, a definition of health would likely constitute the continuation of activities pursued at younger ages or the substitution of new activities in old age.

Personality Theories. Personality theories explain aging in terms of an individual's distinctive behavioral and psychological responses (Birren, 1964), which may be identified by the concept of personality. A basic tenet of *developmental or life cycle theory* (Neugarten, 1964; Lowenthal, 1975) is that people (young or old) are not alike, and that people have their own personalities and styles of living. An individual is said to have aged successfully if he or she maintains a mature, integrated personality while aging, and this is the basis of life satisfaction. Continuity and persistence of personality traits are seen as shaping old age (Neugarten, Havighurst, and Tobin, 1968), which explains the inadequacy of monolithic theoretical frameworks for successful aging (Hendricks and Hendricks, 1981). Public policies consistent with this theoretical school would seek to assist individuals in maintaining continuity in status throughout the life cycle. Social policies would be highly individualized in order to meet each individual's needs, inasmuch as the aging process is characterized by great individual variability (Ragan and Davis, 1978).

Each of these three social and psychological theories seeks an explanation of aging largely in terms of the individual, with the relationship of social structure to aging largely unattended (Dowd, 1980). As a consequence, these theories are of limited utility in explaining how the structural attributes of social class and institutions such as public policy, the economic system, and the medical system affect health and aging in society.

Theory of Age Stratification. A macrosociological approach is taken in the theory of age stratification (Riley, Johnson, and Foner, 1972). This theory explains the "linkages among age, personality, social structure, valued resources and late life involvement" (Hendricks and Hendricks, 1981, p. 130). It posits that the experience of age can be understood along two dimensions in time: the life course cycle, emphasizing the fulfillment of social roles, and the larger historical context of the shared cultural experience of each successive generation. Age-stratification theory is useful in distinguishing and elevating an understanding of the import of age, period, and cohort effects. It is concerned with the effects of the social system on older individuals in terms of role, status, and norms. The policy implications of this theory focus attention on the structured inequalities which are regarded as an intrinsic part of a society organized along a hierarchy of socially defined age strata. Age strata are maintained largely by the social institutions of family, religion, education, and that segment of the economy encompassing tax structure, retirement rules, and public and private sector policy (Ragan and Wales, 1980).

Although the age-stratification theory acknowledges that older persons are systematically disadvantaged in terms of income, work roles, and prestige, it does not examine the issues of equity (distributive justice) and the underlying values governing the distribution of resources, power, and opportunity (Ragan and Wales, 1980). Yet the relevant question is "whether or not all age-related changes operate uniformly for all social classes in a given society" (Hendricks and Hendricks, 1981, p. 131). From the political economy perspective, the shortcomings of the age-stratification model are "its failure to adequately link the effects of class with those of age" (Dowd, 1980, p. 33) and its lack of attention to the political and economic structure as independently affecting aging and health.

Socioenvironmental Theories. Socioenvironmental theories of aging emphasize the interdependence between the aging experience and the social environment within which it occurs. The socioenvironmental orientation encompasses explicit socioenvironmental theory (Gubrium, 1973), ecological theories (Bruhn, 1971), exchange theories (Dowd, 1975), social breakdown theory (Kuypers and Bengtson, 1973), and symbolic interactionist theories (Rose, 1967; Becker, 1963). It calls attention to the potential for the intervention and modification of what many have conceptualized as a unidirectional aging process. Interactions—and the social institutions that create and maintain them—may produce results (for example, confused elderly) that are incorrectly attributed to inevitable biological or psychological processes. Public policy approaches consistent with this orientation would support restructuring the environment that negatively labels older persons, accords them lower exchange value for their resources, or otherwise fosters negative (rather than positive) outcomes in old age.

Conceptual Issues in the Health and Aging Literature. Conceptual issues in the health and aging literature are best summarized by Hickey (1980), who poses an explanatory model utilizing the nature/nurture framework. He develops the concept of *primary aging*, derived from nature, biology, and genetics, and that of *secondary aging*, which is the effect of the environment on development and health in old age. The environment is conceptualized in terms of two dimensions: (1) food, toxicity, chemicals, and stress, and (2) lifestyle and behavior patterns. This latter focus on the link between health status and behavior, social support, and life changes (for example, relocation, retirement, and stress) reflects the general contribution of epidemiology research on health and aging. This literature has made an important contribution in calling attention to the limitations of the biomedical model for poor aged and disabled persons suffering from chronic illness. It is postulated that chronic illness (a physical or mental illness persisting over a long period of time) requires a wholly new approach that treats the social, environmental, and psychological, as well as the biological, aspects of disease (Butler and Newacheck, 1981). The main emphasis of intervention strategy is on modification of individual lifestyles and behavior. Much of the related literature is directed toward improvement of professional skills in the assessment and management of the elderly within institutions and the community (Somers and Fabian, 1981). This literature, however, does not examine the causal links between health status in old age and such macrolevel concerns as economic policy, the structure of the labor force, or the impact of commodity production (Doyal, 1979).

Overall, social gerontologists in the United States have legitimized incremental and individualistic approaches to public policy for the elderly by directing their analyses largely at the individual and social-psychological levels or at the social system level. Their questions and concepts render the economic and political structure residual in explaining old age. The resultant research has therefore predominantly been concerned with social integration and cohort effects and with biomedical and psychological models of aging.

The approaches that have gained ascendancy are reflected in the research priorities of the major federal research institutes. Gerontologists both outside and inside the federal research establishment, particularly the National Institute on Aging, have called for research to unlock the mysteries of the aging process and to distinguish the mutable from the immutable dimensions of aging. In the view of Congress, the public, and powerful segments of the research community, the most promising and popular research is in the biological and biomedical sciences (see Chapter 2). While this is not surprising in view of the way this society tends to think about social problems in general and about aging in particular, the imbalance between research on the biological versus the social origins of the manifestations of old age is likely to prevent a full understanding of the very processes that the research is designed to identify. Old age is, to an as yet unknown degree, shaped by social as well as biological factors.

Similarly, the propensity in this society to think of old age as synonymous with disease is a fallacy widely shared by professionals in the medical establishment. For years, old people have been treated by medical professionals and practitioners who ignore or confuse their health problems with their age. As a result, the health complaints of individual elders are often given a "wastebasket diagnosis" (Butler and Lewis, 1982), especially if and when they involve mental impairment, confusion, or depression. Yet demographic and epidemiological data point to increased longevity and a shift from infectious to chronic diseases. Thus there is an imperative need to disentangle the effects of disease from those of aging and the effects of aging from those of economic and political forces in order to develop a valid, substantive understanding of health and aging and appropriate health policy.

Overview

The significance of the political economy literature is in its directing attention to how the treatment of older people in society and the experience of old age itself are related to an economy whose boundaries are no longer limited to the United States alone but include worldwide economic and political conditions (Amin et al., 1982; Mandel, 1978; Castells, 1980). The task of the political economy of aging is to locate society's treatment of the aged in the context of the economy (national and international), the role of the state, the conditions of the labor market, and the class, sex, race, and age divisions in society. This will require serious consideration of the relationship of capitalism to aging (Myles, 1983). Issues to be examined include the dilemmas and contradictions in maintaining both a market economy and a democracy—that is, in jointly advancing the public interest in a democracy and private profit in a capitalist society.

Politics and economics, although appearing to be abstract concepts, are lived, experienced, and activated through historically and structurally situated conditions and forces. They affect old age. The political economy perspective views the researchable questions about aging and health as structural ones (A. Walker, 1980). The structural approach commences with the proposition that the status, resources, and health of the elderly, and even the trajectory of the aging process itself, are conditioned by one's location in the social structure and the economic and political factors that affect it. Both the health and the dependency of the elderly are to be understood in terms of the labor market and the social relations that the market produces (A. Walker, 1980; 1981). This structural view may be contrasted to individualistic approaches, which give primary emphasis to explaining individual aging, health, and health policy within a given context or structure.

The political economy approach to health and aging calls attention to the following premises:

· The attributional labels applied to the elderly are important in shaping health in old age.
· Health policy and the politics of health mirror societal issues, problems, arrangements, and opportunities (that is, the social structure). As such, health policy reflects the advantages and disadvantages of men and women, of whites and nonwhites, and of skilled and unskilled labor in the society.
· The distribution of health and illness and the organization of health care are also related to these same social arrangements and opportunities, as well as to the distribution of power and influence and the inequalities in that distribution.
· Health policy mirrors the dominant ideologies and belief systems that enforce, bolster, and extend the structure of advantage and disadvantage in the larger social order.
· Health policy and the treatment of the aged as a product of health care policies serve to maintain the economic, political, and social order.
· The social structure shapes how older individuals are perceived and how they perceive themselves and thus shapes their sense of worth and power.

Health policy, viewed in a political economy framework, provides a portrait of the social and political struggles among contending interests and forces in the society.

Chapter

2

Theoretical Perspectives

Health, illness, and health care in old age are directly related to the nature of the society in which they occur. The political economy of health emphasizes the relevance of this context, in terms of the resulting social institutions and social relations, for understanding how health is defined and treated in our society. Health policy in the United States reflects the dominant influence of the society's orientation toward economic growth and private profit. Aging, health, health policy, and health care are all affected by the continual drive for private profit and the accompanying push to reduce the costs of production.

As used here, political economy does not postulate a "one-variable causal model," in which capitalism is seen as the simple cause of everything related to health (Kelman, 1975). However, problems with health and with health policy are to be understood and investigated as being intrinsic to the nature of the social organization in the United States, which is built around private enterprise, private property, and the social relations that result from their pursuit.

The political economy of health and aging draws from two theoretical strands: (1) medical sociology and its critique (Waitzkin and Waterman, 1974; Navarro, 1976) and the emerging political economy of health; and (2) theories of social policy and the welfare state.

Medical Sociology

Initial work in medical sociology reflected concern with practical problem solving for the medical profession and with strategies for dealing with organizational problems (Stacey and Homans, 1978). Much attention has been given to the medical profession, physicians, doctor-patient interactions, and the organization of medicine, while less attention has been paid to the relationships among social structure, social class, and health and illness (Conrad and Kern, 1981). Strauss (1957) has described the dual focus of this field as (a) sociology *in* medicine, which deals with applied problems of doctors and health care delivery systems (for example, hospitals) in order to improve medical practice, and (b) sociology *of* medicine, which focuses on basic sociological research on medicine as a social institution, with physicians remaining at the core of inquiry and nonphysicians seen as adjunct or ancillary (Twaddle, 1982).

The underlying assumptions of much work in medical sociology have been characterized by Doyal (1979) and others (Navarro, 1976; Berliner, 1977; Renaud, 1975) as supporting and legitimizing a medical perspective, as well as the natural sciences as the basis for understanding and treating health. Three assumptions have typified work in the field (Doyal, 1979).

First, health and illness have been considered by medical sociologists largely as *individual* phenomena, and the biological causation of disease is rarely questioned, even when social dimensions are also examined. Because the determinants of health and illness are viewed as biological, "patterns of morbidity and mortality [are seen as having] . . . little to do with the social economic environment in which they occur" (Doyal, 1979, p. 12). This approach to health has directly or indirectly supported the idea that the appropriate or best solutions to improving health lie in increased biomedical research and in the application of biomedically based interventions. This in turn has reinforced the power and legitimacy of the medical profession as the dominant provider of health care for the population, including the elderly.

Second, medicine's claim to being a science has generally been taken as a given, rather than being empirically investigated. Medical interventions have been assumed to be based on an inherently objective scientific method, producing incontrovertibly objective facts. A contrasting approach might be to examine such claims in terms of their ideological content (Navarro, 1976). The medical-scientific approach supports a "mechanistic conception of human beings which sees disturbances at the level of the individual organism and does not seek causes for those disturbances at the level of political and economic systems" (Waitzkin, 1979, p. 696). Medical sociology has largely overlooked the environmental, social, and occupational factors in health and has also ignored the role of health care policies and institutions (for example, the workplace) oriented toward maximizing profit in the production and management of disease in ways that are both profitable and supportive of our capitalist society.

Third, work in medical sociology has proceeded on the assumption that Western scientific medicine is the primary and best means of dealing with disease. This applies both to specific medical interventions and to the institutional organization of medical care. This notion supports the assumption that more biological research and more medical care are what are most needed to improve health. The influence of these assumptions on the literature of health and aging is apparent. The attention to aging as a biophysiological process (see Chapters 1 and 6) and to the measurement of health as a biological and functional state in gerontology reflects the dominance of medical and productivity-oriented concerns.

Twaddle (1982) has argued that medical sociology is moving toward a "sociology of health" characterized by a focus on social systems and institutions, a system-centered conception of prevention, and a critical sociocultural stance relative to health. This movement is in part a result of the "demonstrated . . . limitations of an individualistic approach to health problems" (Twaddle, 1982, p. 353). Some of the reasons given for the shift are

1. developments in medicine itself, such as the increasing alienation of patients from doctors, the theoretical crisis of the germ theory of disease, and the loss of belief in the pure moral character of the medical field and the effectiveness of medicine;
2. competition among health groups and approaches, including alternatives to Western medicine; and
3. sociological developments, such as the emergence of critical and system theories concerned with social structure, social change, and social class.

To a limited extent, these emerging sociological perspectives are reflected in the literature on the political economy of aging (A. Walker, 1980, 1981; Townsend, 1981; Olson, 1982).

This "other face" of medical sociology—the critical stance—is instructive and applicable to our interest in health in old age. Four themes are noteworthy: the stratified nature of health, health care, and health policy; struggles over the definition of health and attention to the social and economic sources of disease; the commodification of health and the corporatization of medical care; and health care and health policy as a form of social control.

Stratification and Health

Waitzkin and Waterman (1974), Friedson (1970a; 1970b), Zola (1975), and others have identified the stratified nature of medicine and medical care as a system of social relationships involving the unequal relations of authority and intimacy, and of dominance and dependency. This stratification extends beyond patient and doctor. It is also reflected in the dominance and legalized monopoly of physicians over nursing and other health professions in the certification of illness and in the right to dispense treatment. Medical stratification validates and reproduces societal inequalities and the structure of disadvantage and advantage among members of the society. Those with low incomes, minorities, and women are unfavorably dealt with both as consumers and as employees in this system. The medical profession's dominance is reflected in health policy for the elderly—both in Medicare and Medicaid. The stratified character of illness, disease, disability, and mortality also has been widely acknowledged (see Chapter 5). That health and income are inversely related has been demonstrated (Conrad and Kern, 1981).

The Definition of Health

Health and illness have been defined in many ways, and the political and economic dimensions of those definitions are relevant here. For example, it is in the interest of a private market economy to define health in terms of one's capacity to be productive (to contribute to profit-making activity), or "functional health." In contrast, it is in the citizen's interest to define health in terms of one's ability to control one's destiny, or "experiential health" (Kelman, 1975). Because of private industry's need for a healthy work force, medicine fulfills an important role in designating treatments for and ameliorating the effects of diseases that have been contracted or hazards to which workers have been exposed in unsafe and unhealthy work environments.

As noted, the significance of the biological definitions and the medical ideology and processing of illness is (a) the shift of responsibility for the problem onto the individual by denying the effects of social or workplace-related factors in illness or disease, and (b) the profitable use of medicine to prevent the widespread recognition of these social origins and thereby to reduce the potential for social disturbance that an aware, sick, and dissatisfied populace of any age could represent.

The tendencies in our society to link aging with diseases, to think of aging as a biological process of decline (see Chapter 1), and to equate old age with the need for medical care similarly place aging squarely within the domain of medical treatment. The resulting medicalization of old age is costly to the individual and to the public. It also shifts attention from the societal dimensions of health in aging, such as enforced economic dependency for millions through mandatory retirement, to the biological dimensions of health and the treatment of individuals through services that are delivered at a profit.

The Commodification of Health

The medical-engineering model of health and illness, which dominates public policy, posits a rational system of endogenous causes within the context of the body's cellular and biochemical systems (Renaud, 1975). The ascendance of the engineering approach to improving health dates back to the seventeenth century (Powles, 1973). Such a strategy supports society's growing investment in medical care as the primary determinant of good health (McKeown, 1978). A broader conception of health would also emphasize the importance of social, economic, and political factors in determining the health of populations (Andreano and Weisbrod, 1974). Indeed, as Arrow has observed, the "causal factors in health are many, and the provision of medical care is only one" (1963, p. 941).

The most important political consequence of the wholesale adoption of the medical-engineering model is that it transforms health needs into commodities for specific economic markets. It supports high technology, manufacture of drugs, and specialization by experts who treat parts of the problem presented by "consumers" seeking goods and services in the medical marketplace. Most of all, this paradigm obscures the extent to which illness is determined by exogenous causes. In contrast, the ecological approach to health would stress that humans are biological and social beings in relation to the entire political and social ecosystem (Renaud, 1975). The medical-engineering model of health and illness and its commodification of health have shaped contemporary health policy for older persons. This approach is compatible with the treatment, quality of care, and incentives in the organization and delivery of health care in the United States.

The first boost to the commodification of health came in 1946 with the passage of the Hill-Burton legislation, which subsidized the private sector for construction and expansion of hospital facilities. Later, with the passage of Medicare and Medicaid in the mid-1960s, the long-term financial needs of the health care industry were secured. Often this did not result directly in profits but rather in the financial underwriting of extravagantly technical and expensive medical centers with newly acquired facilities, specialties, research, and technology. The passage of such major legislation providing federal funds to support hospital construction (Hill-Burton) and health services to the elderly (Medicare) and to the poor (Medicaid) has been described as a "gold rush" for the modern hospital center (Ehrenreich and Ehrenreich, 1971). The Ehrenreichs called the health industry a big, profitable, and booming business, with government guaranteed markets, and a medical-industrial complex. Health has come to be viewed as a commodity for private investment and profit-making ventures. Ehrenreich and Ehrenreich (1971) considered the "American health empire" to be composed of lucrative industries in drugs, hospital supplies and equipment, health insurance, nursing homes, and hospitals, with unknown billions of dollars of after-tax profits. Government subsidization of the market has included health manpower legislation, hospital construction, tax deductions for medical expenses, tax exemptions to nonprofit hospitals, funding for basic biological and chemical research, and Medicare and Medicaid. Ehrenreich and Ehrenreich described the future as portending increased corporatization and profits.

In 1980, Relman described a "new medical industrial complex"— a $35 to $40 billion industry characterized by overuse and fragmentation of services, undue emphasis on technology, screening for profitable patients and services, and inappropriate influence on national health policy. Relman's primary concern was the shift of service provision and control from nonprofit institutions and physicians to profit-making industries and corporations. According to Relman, this shift represents the weakening of the "best kind of regulation of the health care market place . . . the informed judgments of physicians working in the interests of their patients" (1980, p. 967).

What is most relevant to our concern with health and aging is that "business and government have begun to look at medical care as more nearly an economic product than a social good" (Iglehart, 1982, p. 120). Within this context, the incentive is to maximize profits rather than health. The consequence for the elderly, for all persons dependent on public policy and programs, is that social needs are turned into profit-making commodities (Scull, 1977). The needs of the elderly are defined and processed by the medical industry in ways that merely serve to medicalize old age further and to exacerbate rather than alleviate the dependency of the elderly. The creation of what has been called "the aging enterprise" (Estes, 1979) reflects one aspect of this trend.

Health Care as a Form of Social Control

Social control "is usually conceptualized as the means by which society secures adherence to social norms; specifically, how it minimizes, eliminates, or normalizes deviant behavior" (Conrad and Schneider, 1980, p. 7). A sociopolitical analysis focuses on the social control functions of the medical system—that is, the structure and organization of health care delivery. One way in which health care acts as a system of social control is by the authority of physicians to define an individual's problem and prescribe solutions. The dominance of physicians, a professional elite composed largely of white upper-class males, in physician-client relationships "can only act to promote acquiescence to a social system built on class and sex-based inequalities" (Ehrenreich and Ehrenreich, 1974, p. 35).

The Ehrenreichs have identified two types of social control of health care that are applicable to health policy for the aging: disciplinary and cooptative. The organization and structure of health policy provides *disciplinary control* by limiting access to care for the poor elderly. Limitations in Medicaid coverage include inequity and inadequacy in coverage from state to state and stringency in eligibility requirements. These limitations influence the health-seeking behavior of the elderly poor and demonstrate to them that society will not solve their problems if they have failed in the labor market. *Cooptative control* applies to the middle-income elderly, who could easily become impoverished without the basic coverage of Medicare. Having access to the guaranteed benefits of Medicare, these elderly are not inclined to "rock the boat" by demanding major national health insurance or other reforms. In accepting the health care that is provided, both poor and middle-income elderly (and society) become increasingly dependent on a highly profitable, technologically and scientifically based medical approach, which views and treats health in old age predominantly along biological/disease dimensions.

Theories of Social Policy and the Welfare State

Four theoretical paradigms are relevant to the analysis of social policy in health and aging: liberal political theory, pluralist theory, elite theory, and class theory. Each approach postulates different explanations of how public policy is formed, how different elements of society are taken into account, and how public policy is changed. Each reflects a different perspective on the classic sociological question of social order—how society and its institutions, such as health care, are held together.

One major dimension crosscutting these theories is the extent to which each postulates that the social order (and the dominant institutions) may be explained by consensus or conflict. The *consensus approach* posits that society is held together by shared values and because people in the society generally agree with the way things are organized and functioning (Parsons, 1951). Such a perspective argues that medical institutions, for example, are the way they are because members of society agree that they should be that way. Institutions such as the state are held to be neutral and operating in the universal interests of all elements of society. A contrasting view of society is the *conflict approach*—that the social order is held together by the dominance of some over others. The outcomes of conflict and power struggles explain how society is organized and functions. Society is viewed as being held together by constraint—not by consensus (Collins, 1968). Medical institutions are organized the way they are because some are able to impose their ideas, interests, and policies on others. From this viewpoint, the state tends to be seen not as a neutral arbiter of the public interest, but rather as a reflection in various forms of the interests of those who are most powerful. Similarly, medical care organization and health policy reflect the outcomes of power struggles and benefit the factions that dominate resources such as money, ideas, and political organization.

The liberal political theory and the pluralist theory emerge from the consensus tradition, while the elite and class theories reflect the conflict tradition. In this book, the political economy perspective draws from the conflict model of society and builds on the elite and class theories. A review of all four theories will clarify our approach.

Liberal Political Theory. Liberal political theory emphasizes individual rights and a limited role for government in the interest of political and economic freedom. Welfare economics and government policy are delimited as being appropriate (1) when goods and services cannot be individually consumed but benefit all members (for example, defense), or (2) to compensate for the effect of external factors that may harm or benefit one party or another in the production or consumption process (Gough, 1979). The unrestrained operation of the capitalist market is theorized to maximize "welfare," except under limited circumstances (Friedman, 1962). Except under these circumstances, the state should not intervene in the allocation of resources. The theory holds that the distribution of resources is proportionate to one's contribution. The consensus of all members of society and the overall benefits they receive support the continued operation of the market-dominated economy.

Pluralist Theory. Pluralist theory (also called interest group theory) posits that power is widely diffused in Western democracies such as the United States. This political market perspective holds that competition between interest groups is a positive feature of society and that different groups interact essentially on an equal footing; thus there is overt denial that any single group or class is a dominant force in the society (Dahl, 1956).

Research from this perspective has focused on the influence of organized interest groups in competition for scarce resources (Dahl, 1956) and the lobbying in Congress by such groups to promote their solutions to problems and to obtain resources (Cater and Lee, 1972). The influence of medical and hospital lobbies and professional groups in shaping public policy to serve their economic and political interests has been studied extensively (Feldstein, 1977; Law, 1974; Marmor, 1970; Alford, 1976). In characterizing the process by which decisions are made, the focus of analysis tends to be on the "actors" in the political arena and the interest groups they represent. The government tends to be seen as a neutral arbiter whose role is to facilitate and, when necessary, mediate the competition between interest groups. However, the "political market approach cannot explain why there is a welfare state, nor why the U.S. version of the welfare state is different from that of other industrial countries" (Dunham and Marmor, 1978, p. 278).

Pluralist theory venerates interest groups as a positive source of democratic participation, whereas conflict perspectives question whether interest groups represent the pubic interest or fulfill democratic principles. Conflict theories note that many sectors of society are not represented by interest groups and that interest group politics are concerned with immediate gains for special interests. The pluralist perspective ignores the large-scale vested interests that dominate the policy-making process and shape public programs. According to conflict theory, U.S. public policy in health and aging both reflects and serves dominant structural interests built into the operation of our society's major legal, economic, medical, and social institutions (Estes, 1979; Alford, 1976). Pluralist theory, on the other hand, contends that health policy for the aged is the result of an essentially fair process of accommodation among competing interests for scarce public resources.

Elite Theory. Elite theory, based on the work of Max Weber (1946), C. Wright Mills (1956), Floyd Hunter (1953) and others, posits that public policy and the allocation of resources result from conflict and power struggles, in which certain groups and organizations dominate the resources and control the outcomes. The major types of resources in power struggles over health or any other issue are (1) ideas and beliefs, (2) economic (material) resources, and (3) political resources, such as control of the appropriate bureaucratic apparatus or political organization. Conflict is seen as inevitable and continuous; it creates the dynamics for possible social change. The dominance of certain groups and interests (elites) through their positions in major social institutions, rather than the consensus of disparate members of the society, determines the stability of the organization of health care and of other aspects of our social system. The distribution of power is seen as being directly related to the dominant elites, and as reflecting more or less their interests in public policy (Whitt, 1979).

Class Theory. Class theory sees a relationship between the organization of society, including its institutions, such as governmental structure and medicine, and the distribution of wealth or control of the production process. The political process shaping policy outcomes is understood in terms of institutional structure and the relation of social classes to one another. The structure of social institutions, and particularly of the economy, is seen as placing major limits on the behavior of individuals and groups in society (Whitt, 1979). Theorists working within this perspective contend that in capitalist societies there is a dominant class and that it is this class that controls the means of production.

Since production is largely controlled by profit-making corporations, most people are dependent on the capitalist economy and the wage and salary income provided through it. Class theory argues that power accrues to the dominant class because of this control over the production of wealth, but this power is not seen as absolute, because political and economic tensions prevent or limit the dominant class from acting solely in its own interest. Social institutions, such as medicine, and the social policies supporting them, such as Medicare, are examined in terms of how they address the interests of different classes. According to class theory, social, economic, and cultural institutions are biased in the way they operate and in how they shape the agenda of public and private issues and our thinking about them. The link between the economically and politically dominant classes is of interest. Navarro (1976) has called attention to class relations underlying the delivery of health care in the United States. Others have focused on the welfare state as a necessary outgrowth of the needs of capitalist societies.

Theory of the State

What is the state, and how does it function? Broadly speaking, the term "the state" is used to denote the major social and economic institutions in society, including the executive, legislative, and judicial branches of government, the military, the criminal justice system, educational institutions, and public health and welfare institutions (Waitzkin, 1983). Although there are many theories of the state (Offe and Ronge, 1982; Frankel, 1982; O'Connor, 1973; Gough, 1979), most theorists would agree with Weber that "the first role of any state is to assure the survival of the economic system" (cited in Navarro, 1975b, p. 86).

Throughout this book, the term is largely concerned with that portion of the state—the government—responsible for shaping modern welfare institutions. Government affects these institutions by virtue of its power to allocate and distribute scarce resources to ensure the survival and growth of the economy, to mediate between different segments and classes of society, and to ameliorate social conditions that could threaten the existing order. Ultimately, the state is an instrument of violence, empowered to use force in order to maintain the social order (Weber, 1946). Since the state is the most powerful organized instrument in society, it is important to study the struggles to control it because they illuminate the distribution of resources and shape of power in the society.

Offe and Ronge (1982) have identified four characteristics of the state in capitalist societies: (1) property is private, and privately owned capital is the basis of the economy; (2) resources generated through private profit and the growth of private wealth indirectly finance the state (for example, through taxation); (3) the state is thereby "dependent on a source of income which it does not itself organize . . . thus [it] has a general 'interest' in facilitating" the growth of private profit in order to perpetuate itself (Giddens and Held, 1982, p. 192); and (4) in democracies such as the United States, political elections and the expression of the voice of an electorate disguise the basic fact that the resources available for distribution by the state are dependent on the success of private profit and capital reinvestment, not on the will of the electorate. A fifth attribute of the state in capitalist societies is its accountability for the success of the economy; the state bears the brunt of public dissatisfaction with an unhealthy economy. These attributes particularly create problems for the democratic capitalist state. Myles (1984) has questioned whether it is inherently contradictory for the state to jointly advance the interests of private capital, with the need to ensure private profit and reinvestment, and the interests of a democratic society, with its pressures for equality and redistributive functions of the state to mediate the inequities and displacement created by a market-based economy.

As O'Connor (1973) has argued, the state in U.S. society has two major functions. First, the state ensures the conditions favorable to economic growth and private profit (allowing for the accumulation of wealth). Second, the state ensures the continuing legitimacy and operation of the social order by alleviating those conditions and problems generated by the free enterprise system (such as unemployment) that might create destructive social unrest. This is accomplished through the provision of publicly subsidized benefits. One problem is that both of these functions of the state require the expenditure of public resources. State expenditures associated with accumulation meet the needs of business and industry through favorable tax treatment and government subsidies for building industrial parks, for educating and transporting the labor force, and for other investments (such as highways and sewers) that lower production costs. State expenditures for what is traditionally referred to as social welfare reflect the displacement costs of the operation of our economic system—the costs in poverty, sexism, racism, and ageism.

The tension created by the demand for these two types of expenditures often results in a propensity for the state to spend itself into fiscal crisis. This creates its own consequences in the state's necessary retreat from the fiscal underwriting of the costs of one or both of these functions. Furthermore, as capitalist industry gets larger and more monopolistic in character, moves into international markets, and is more technologically advanced, the costs of capital formation and reinvestment increase. At the same time, there are increased demands on the state for assistance in meeting those costs (tax subsidies, roads, bridges, toxic waste clean-ups, etc.). While the state subsidizes more of the costs, the benefits of the investments continue to be returned as private profit. Furthermore, since monopoly is not labor intensive, it pushes people into a diminishing competitive sector. This exacerbates unemployment and increases the need for state subsidies to alleviate the cumulative negative consequences of these processes. From a political economy perspective, the dual functions of public spending are of the utmost importance because one sees the size of the federal budget not only in nominal terms but also in terms of the complex interaction between the public and private sectors of the economy.

Analyses of public policy directing the allocation and distribution of resources for our nation's older citizens need to go beyond the scarcity model. It is not merely a question of whether there are enough resources to support domestic social spending. A more important issue is the impact of allocating an increasing share of resources to the aged on business and economic growth and on the relations of industry and labor (Myles, 1984). The essential issue, from a political economy perspective, concerns the effect public spending has on the functions of the private economy in terms of ensuring and maintaining a flow of capital for profits and investments. Conservative economists, for example, have charged that Social Security has reduced the public's reliance on the market, increased the individual's dependency on government, and reduced incentives for personal savings, which are a major source of the investment capital essential for economic growth (Rahn and Simonson, 1980). The economic significance of the "graying of America" is that:

> It increases the size of the public economy and reduces the share of the national income directly subject to market forces. Thus, while population aging is unlikely to break the "national bank" it will alter the bank's structure of ownership and control. (Myles, 1982, p. 19)

Ultimately, how many resources are controlled by the state or by the private economy is a political decision. The relative amounts allocated to supporting the supply of capital (for reinvestment and profit) and to workers or to social welfare costs are never set, but are constantly subject to political and economic struggle. Domestic social spending for income and health needs competes not only with corporate and business growth but also with other political priorities, namely, defense spending.

Under the U.S. economic system, economic growth and private profit occur only when capital is invested in labor, materials, and production facilities. Labor produces commodities, and these commodities are sold on markets for amounts greater than the capital invested (that is, the original investment must be realized, and some surplus must be realized as profit). The markets for commodities are composed of consumption based on earnings (that is, capital invested in labor) and investment in materials and productive facilities, particularly the former. Thus the market depends largely on employment and earnings in the process of production.

The profits from the production process depend not only on the costs of labor as expressed in wages, but also on other costs and on the rate of productivity. Therefore, how much is produced and the conditions under which it is produced are issues of continual struggle. Lower costs of production and demands for higher productivity may result in working conditions that have a deleterious effect on the welfare and health status of workers. Moreover, government itself plays a role in allocating a major portion of the economic surplus (through taxation, creation of debt, etc.), and governmental expenditures also affect the rate of profit (accumulation) and the ability of workers and the public to purchase or consume products (consumption). Government policies may also transfer profits and consumption from one group or class to another.

The application of the political economy approach to the health of the elderly requires two avenues of inquiry. One is an elaboration of our previous consideration of the relationship of state spending to the maintenance of economic growth and to the welfare of the elderly. The other involves questions of class relations, especially those involving the aged.

Social Spending, Economic Growth, and the Elderly

Social spending can perform a number of functions: (1) ensuring a supply of productive labor, (2) creating effective demand for goods and services, (3) ameliorating conditions that might be politically threatening, (4) legitimating the state and the economic system, and (5) controlling social behavior. Social spending is constrained in that it must not be allowed to undermine the supply of productive labor, divert too much from private enterprise, or create new political instabilities or underwrite policies or organize actions that may challenge the system. Government spending is clearly related to the function of ensuring a supply of productive and healthy labor. State spending has been drawn into programs of education, training, nutrition, shelter and health care for at least a portion of the young in order to provide a productive labor force. Also, programs such as unemployment compensation have ensured the continued supply of labor at different skill levels through times when such labor is not needed by the economy (workers are not technically required to accept jobs at lower skill levels, although economic necessity may nevertheless drive many to do so). The aged may have needs similar in many ways to these other age groups, but they relate differently to the functions and limitations of social spending.

Social spending on the elderly in the form of income programs, especially Social Security retirement benefits, has ensured that most older workers leave the labor force. The majority of retired persons, who are dependent on Social Security, are further discouraged from working by the 50 percent cut in retirement benefits for every dollar earned over a low base figure. Nevertheless, the aged are not entirely removed from the labor market; in 1980, about 20 percent of males aged 65 or over continued in the labor force (U.S. Bureau of the Census, 1982). Thus it appears that, even though the assurance of retirement is an important function of labor market maintenance by the state (Graebner, 1980; Myles, 1984), the aged cannot be written off entirely as participants in that market.

It is an axiomatic principle of public welfare that benefits cannot be too generous or they might undermine the incentive of the broad populace to work. On this count, however, the aged can be expected to be considered as legitimate recipients of welfare state spending—they are, by and large, outside the labor force, and many social policies are structured as *disincentives* for the aged to work. Moreover, the existence of benefits for the aged, pegged to a work history, can be seen as further inducement for the younger population to work up until the day of retirement. However, benefits to the aged cannot be limitless. First, the revenue for benefits is largely derived from the wages of the working population and therefore cannot exceed the growth in real wages. If it does, the ability of workers to save or to consume (the incentive to work) may be undermined. Moreover, benefits to the aged may in part draw on resources that might otherwise be allocated to economic growth (for example, capital formation).

Of course, social spending may create considerable effective demand. To some degree, this works through transfers from one sector to another. For example, middle-income earners are taxed and payments are made to the poor. In this case effective demand is only transferred from one place to another, in part from one market to another. The concern of supply-side economists is that social spending increases consumption rather than stimulates investment, in order to ensure economic growth.

Direct social spending, such as public funding of a "social industrial complex" (O'Connor, 1973) or, more specifically, an "aging enterprise" (Estes, 1979), has another connection to the economy. When the government becomes directly or indirectly the purchaser of health or social services, many of these commodities (for example, nursing home care) are produced by and purchased from the private sector. The health care industry (the medical-industrial complex) in particular has been an industry with a rapidly expanding investment. In health care, investments (especially in the case of reinvestment by hospitals) are often made to build the status and dominance of medical institutions, rather than to make the most profitable investment in strict economic terms. Thus, although health care institutions may derive profit from their activities and reinvest it, the investments may not be subject to the requirements of profit maximization operating in other sectors of the economy. As an example, hospitals may tend to overinvest in beds they cannot fill, and the resulting low occupancy rates then represent an unproductive use of capital. Such overinvestment may then threaten the financial viability of the hospital. Hospitals may be able to recoup their investments through both cost-plus reimbursement from government social welfare programs such as Medicare and increases in their rates to private payers, who are increasingly backed by third-party insurers drawing on untaxed health insurance benefits. These forms of return on investment have been accompanied by the escalation of health care costs at two to three times the rate of inflation. That these expenditures are now considered a drain on the economy can be seen in recent legislative attempts to impose prospective and other negotiated health care payments on government programs, to tax health care premiums paid by employers, and to restructure the health care industry by favoring health maintenance organizations (HMO's) and other competitive modes of health care delivery.

Insofar as investment in the health care industry draws funds from other industries, the problem is heightened. For example, health benefits constitute a large part of the fringe benefits paid by industries such as auto and steel to their workers; they are estimated by some to cost as much as $3,000 per U.S. automobile produced. Escalating health care costs and insurance premiums increase costs to industry and reduce profits. Likewise, the health care industry competes with other industries for funds by incurring large long-term debts.

The key argument of the opposition to social spending is that it reduces the support of the system of private enterprise, draining funds away from private investment and thus from economic growth. Income transfers to the aged, particularly Social Security benefits, have been described by conservative economists as siphoning off funds from "productive uses," drawing on funds that could otherwise be available for investment capital or for consumption by younger people. Likewise, the aging enterprise can be seen as "too expensive" to ensure continuing growth and profit in the economy. This position is particularly defensible because health care costs, which are second only to income programs in terms of public spending for the aged, have been increasing faster than has inflation in other areas of the economy.

Social spending on the aged may fulfill a number of purposes at once, including altruistic ones. The amelioration of conditions created in consequence of the economic system is one recognized function of the state. Millions of the elderly living in poverty could be politically threatening; the elderly are part of our families, and we expect to grow old ourselves. Moreover, the aged form a vocal constituency through national organizations and interest groups. Finally, the problems of the aged are viewed as the natural consequences of aging and thus perhaps deserving of amelioration.

However, certain forms of social spending may engender conflict within the system. The War on Poverty measures of the 1960s, which mandated political involvement of the poor, were eliminated when they were seen to be threatening to local power structures. In a similar manner, politicians may perceive legal services or advocacy by agencies receiving governmental grants as threatening to the social stability of "business as usual." Given the potential for political conflict, it is not surprising that social spending emphasizes the purchase of institutional and agency services rather than the provision of more adequate income, or recipient-controlled services. The isolation of the problems of aging from those of other groups also diminishes the threat of political conflict by creating divisions between the elderly and the natural allies of the elderly—other socially oppressed groups.

These considerations help to clarify the legitimacy of the aged as "truly needy." Because the aged are not in general part of the labor market, their incentives to work cannot be undermined. There are advantages and disadvantages to social spending, however. Increased funding for social welfare programs may divert funds from support of economic growth. This may be partially offset by funding an aging enterprise or a medical-industrial complex that includes a large private sector. However, this response transfers profit from one industry to another. From the viewpoint of the system, such a transfer may divert funds from basic industry to the hospital and nursing home industries (in large part through private health plans, but also through government spending), and in ways deleterious to economic growth. Thus there are opposing forces working to build up and then to constrain the public costs of an aging enterprise.

Social Class and the Elderly

Wright (1978) has defined the major processes comprising class relations as "control over investments and resources," "control over the physical means of production," and "control over the labor power of others." The political economic concept of class is not limited to what members of different classes derive from the system in the way of income and other resources. In particular, class analysis is concerned with relative control over policy, over resources, and over other people. Moreover, such an approach to class links differences found by class back to the system producing the class divisions. Guillemard has referred to this as a "genetic definition of class positions that links them directly to the social mechanisms by which they are generated" (1982, p. 228).

The concept of class and how it relates specifically to the aged is an important area of inquiry. According to Giddens (1975), there is widespread confusion and ambiguity in the use of the term "class." This seems particularly so for some who have attempted an analysis of the aged and class (Dowd, 1980; Atchley, 1981). In the United States, aging policy is partially based on the assumption that the aged are a separate, distinct class. This approach treats the aged as a dependent group of individuals separate from the productive sector of the economy. In this sense, class refers to the aged as a social group whose members share one common denominator: they are all over 65 years of age and retired or soon to be summoned into retirement. Such a policy, which fosters age-segregated programs and services, is likely to enhance both the dependency status of the aged and intergenerational conflict (Estes, 1979). Moreover, such social policy does not deal seriously with class and other social differences and inequities among the elderly. Income differences are treated unidimensionally as differences in ability to pay. This sets off the "truly needy" from those who can pay, at least in part, for services as commodities. What is not addressed is the larger class implications of aging policies, the differential implications of those policies for different classes among the aged, and the functions of aging policies for the society and its organization as a whole.

One problem in relating Marxist class theory to the aged, according to Dowd (1980), is that the aged are no longer in the productive sector of the economy. Yet this is precisely the critical point of examination for a political economy approach (Guillemard, 1974; 1983; Townsend, 1981; A. Walker, 1980; 1981). Many have observed that the economic inequality and dependency status of the aged are a result of forced retirement and inadequate benefits. The structural dependency of the aged arises from conditions in the labor market and in the stratification and organization of work and society. A. Walker (1981) has argued that it is not age itself that determines retirement, but the socially constructed relationships among age, the division of labor, and the labor market. Retirement itself must be seen as an institution arising from economic forces in society, not as an inevitable obstacle to well-being—as a consistent phenomenon faced in the same way by all members of society, not as a historical barrier suspending the preretirement class structure of society.

Class analysis allows us to consider the differential implications of retirement and old age for each class, as well as the implications of retirement and old age for class relationships. Preretirement class status is a major factor affecting postretirement conditions. Guillemard (1982, p. 226) has discussed "typical life trajectories" related to each class position. However, class relationships may be different in general for the aged from what they are for younger people. This is true in part because of retirement and in part because of a wider disattachment of the aged from the productive process and from society in general and the treatment of the aged as a group apart from society, with different needs from those of other social groups. The fact that most elderly live on fixed incomes is itself both a reflection of class relations and an important factor to consider in any analysis of class and aging. Class analysis of aging therefore presents different problems from a more general analysis of the class dynamics of society; however, the class theory needed to account for the situation of the aged may throw light on class analysis in general. A class analysis of aging may be especially pertinent to what a society based on private enterprise defines as nonproductive groups.

Ehrenreich and Ehrenreich (1979) have proposed a definition of class that, even though it may be problematical in explaining the dynamics of capitalism, promises to be useful in explaining class dynamics involving the aged. In addition to defining class in terms of a "common relation to the economic foundations of society," the Ehrenreichs see class as being

> characterized by a coherent social and cultural existence; members of a class share a common life style, educational background, kinship networks, consumption patterns, work habits, and beliefs. (1979, p. 11)

This definition may be of special importance to the analysis of class and age because it is concerned with dynamics that are still operating among those elders who are no longer in the workplace. In particular, it helps clarify the relationships of working-class aged with the agents of public and private social welfare bureaucracies. Although the Ehrenreichs noted that there is no simple way to define class for some categories of professional workers as a group, certain professional-client relationships can be seen as inherently class relationships.

The processes of detachment from work life operate differently for the aged of different classes, with accompanying variation in the degree to which older individuals are devalued. Retirement separates retirees from whatever control over actual work processes that they might have had, from control over others, and in some cases even from ownership. For example, in medical partnerships, the physician's share must be returned upon retirement. Although the income of a relatively advantaged class location may continue after retirement, the control usually does not. According to Wright's reasoning (1978), the ownership of wealth without effective control over investment and the physical means of production leaves even the wealthy elderly on the periphery of the class dynamics of the larger society. Nevertheless, control that accompanies ownership is less subject to change with old age than is control that stems purely from occupational function. The loss of control with retirement, and its differential loss by class, has important implications for the aged. We need to examine whether those who had some degree of control have either skills or status that is transferable to postretirement activities. The postretirement implications for elders whose histories are characterized by subordination rather than control also must be examined.

These considerations are especially important given Langer and Rodin's (1976) linking of "perceived control" over one's life to survival rates and health status in nursing homes. Even if one accepts Langer's (1981) argument that it is not control but activity averting reduction to "mindlessness" that results in better health, the implications are important to the aged who lose social functions at retirement.

It has been argued (Estes, 1979) that public policy has created an "aging enterprise," with this outcome: "the aged are often processed and treated as a commodity." The bureaucracies, industries, and professionals constituting this enterprise ensure the dependency of the aged on their services and on the maintenance of the class relationships fostered by those services (Sjoberg, Brymer, and Farris, 1966). This dependency is a unilateral one in which bureaucratic structures "and the middle class bureaucrats by whom services usually are delivered, are the medium for interaction between members of lower social classes and the general society" (Estes, 1979, p. 24). This system also tends to isolate the aged from society, largely through age-segregated policies.

Overview

A complete view of class and age, then, must consider a number of dynamics. Being old in the capitalist world is characterized by a detachment from the work process. Retirement alters class dynamics by removing the aged from the immediate relations and functions of the workplace. These relations, however, continue to "live" as a part of the individual retiree's personal history and in the relationships among retirees with common work histories, to the extent of even affecting postretirement life expectancy (Guillemard, 1983). Nevertheless, detachment from work life may mean that the relations of the workplace do not constitute the primary dynamic of class relations for the aged. Ownership of property and access to means of income continue to be sources of class division among the aged.

Any analysis of class and age must concern itself with how the elderly, whatever their previous background, are made dependent by the economic and political organization of society and with how public policy treats the elderly according to their differential preretirement class status. The devaluation of the elderly through work detachment and the physical and mental consequences of their being labeled by society as nonproductive and sick also require examination, in the context of the effects of class of origin and class of destination.

Chapter

3

Historical Perspective on Health Policy and Programs for Older Persons

This chapter is an interpretation of a century of events surrounding the formation of the welfare state and public policies and programs for the aged. Special attention is given to class relations and class struggle and the primary beliefs and values that clashed against new ideas. Two themes emerge from this examination: the class basis of policies and the commodification of health. These themes provide a perspective for exploring the evolution of a stratified system of health care for the elderly and the consequences of this system. Both the highly stratified medical orientation of policies and the commodification of the needs of the elderly meet the requirements of the political economy of the United States.

Many cultural, demographic, and sociopolitical changes have shaped the evolution of U.S. public policies and programs for the elderly. Large-scale economic trends and political events at both the national and international levels have had great import for health policy. Factors such as the rate of economic growth, inflation, labor force trends, and wages produced the conditions and political climate conducive to the expansion or contraction of the welfare state. However, public policy did not simply respond to the objective facts. Choices, often difficult and involving competing and contradictory aims, had to be made. Social and health policies have followed a definite course of action or direction brought about by many political decisions. Policy has often been guided by immediate, practical concerns of the state as well as by individual motives for profit and gain.

Social movements arising before the Depression were important forces in public policy decisions. Influenced by the developing

European social welfare, U.S. efforts for the elderly were organized not on the basis of age but rather on the basis of other issues relevant to the elderly. Examples include the social insurance movement in 1911, which worked toward establishing the "right" of workers to protection against loss of wages due to disability or illness; the mother pension movement of 1915, which worked toward the "right" of poor mothers to raise their children at home rather than send them to institutions; and the trade union movement, which worked toward the "rights" of workers to income security, job opportunities, and safety protection. In the 1920s, the Townsend movement worked toward the "right" of older persons to receive income security and public pensions. This had an enormous influence on developing public support and understanding of the need for future security for retired persons and the role of the government in that need. In the 1960s, the civil rights movement and the women's movement focused on discrimination, inequality of opportunity, and poverty in the United States. These movements served as catalysts for efforts to legislate a national policy on aging and to dramatize the socio-economic conditions of the aged as a distinct and separate group in U.S. society (Estes, 1979). The federal role in domestic social problems, especially in areas of civil rights, medical care, education, and poverty, expanded. Significant efforts were made to improve the well-being of older citizens through social policy. The intervention measures of the Johnsonian era of the 1960s were part of a period of enormous political upheaval, protest, and idealism for effecting change at the national level.

The political outcomes of social reform activists throughout history, however, have been tempered by the needs of capital and the polity. It is widely acknowledged in the literature that mandatory retirement and the pensions to support it were interventional measures developed during the 1930s in relation to the needs of capital for industrial development (Graebner, 1980). The measures also filled the needs of the president to maintain the legitimacy of government by responding to the cataclysmic societal events set off by the Depression. The Social Security Act of 1935 did not represent a national commitment to eradicating dependency in old age so much as an effort to moderate the dependency of the aged in ways that were compatible with the political economy and the need to get the country back on its feet economically.

Ideology and the Welfare State

Public policies affecting the elderly directly or indirectly are the product of an intense political and economic struggle over the past century of U.S. history. This struggle has shaped a welfare state in some ways peculiar to the United States. While many European countries were developing the foundations for a modern welfare state between the 1880s and the 1920s, the idea of social welfare had a much slower rate of acceptance in the United States. Indeed, it took the Depression in the 1930s to translate the idea of social insurance (that is, the welfare state) into real programs compatible with U.S. ideology and economy. In analyzing the formation of the U.S. welfare state, Skocpol and Ikenberry define the modern welfare state as "the emergence and maturation of public programs of social insurance intended to cover risks to a national population from work-injuries, sickness and disability, diminution of earnings in old age, and unemployment" (1982, p. 2). The development of the modern welfare state—especially since World War II—often reflected the "ideals of guaranteed national-minimal provision for the needs of all citizens, in effect melding together security and welfare aid" (Skocpol and Ikenberry, 1982, p. 4). In reality, however, the welfare state in the United States has been characterized by a distinct division between social security and welfare. This, in turn, laid the foundation for the development of a stratified system of health care for older persons.

Public usage of the term "welfare state" emerged in Britain at the time of that country's involvement in World War II. The political philosophy of the welfare state, according to T. H. Marshall, was "born in an atmosphere of confusion" (1964, p. 262). The finer details of what the welfare state ought to encompass and provide to those in need were not clearly agreed on by the different political factions. However, one clear goal of the emerging British welfare state was to eradicate the Elizabethan Poor Law of 1601 and thereby move away from the stigmatizing pauper category to a system incorporating people "in the general body of the free and independent working class, protected and sustained by their basic rights as citizens" (Marshall, 1964, p. 263).

In the United States, the way of dealing with the poor and unemployed was originally modeled after the English Poor Law (Williamson, 1982), which provided a subsistence level of economic relief to the poorest segments and outcasts of society. Elderly persons who were poor or bereft of family were included in the relief policies simply because there were no other special provisions for their care. The primary method of assistance was aid given in the home, known as "outdoor relief." By the nineteenth century this was replaced with "indoor relief," designating the charity-run almshouse, or workhouse, as the means of providing assistance. This shift to the workhouse as a precondition of assistance marked a more restrictive relief policy. The workhouse basically acted as a disincentive to those seeking aid because more often than not residence in a workhouse was accompanied by a loss of dignity, autonomy, and control characteristic of such punitive institutional environments. It was thought that consigning the elderly to the workhouse would put more pressure on family members, especially children, to support their parents in their old age and to plan for their own future by personal savings and thrift (Williamson, 1982). On a macropolitical level, these poor laws were aimed at controlling social unrest attendant to widespread poverty and unemployment. Between the fourteenth and nineteenth century, the laws fluctuated between a predominant policy of repression and one of liberalization, depending on the requirements of the economy, social rebellion, and crimes against property (Williamson, 1982).

The evolution of welfare policy in the United States was complicated by the historical relations among the federal, state, and local governments. Up until the Depression and the New Deal of the 1930s, the guiding principle was the concept of dual federalism—strict separation of power and authority between the federal and state and local governments. During the early years of the Republic, the federal role in domestic social policy was minimal. The one exception to this was the federally funded pension system for veterans of the Civil War and widows and dependents of deceased soldiers (Skocpol and Ikenberry, 1982). Dual federalism (1861–1930s) stressed the independence of each level of government from the others, with the central government concentrating mainly on foreign policy, the military, and monetary and banking areas (D. Walker, 1981). Responsibility for the health and welfare of citizens was left primarily to the discretion of state and local governments. Social welfare benefits were also an essential part of the politicians' trade of bestowing benefits on the poor or sick as small tokens of concern (Skocpol and Ikenberry, 1982).

The evolution of state aid to the poor was gradual. Until New York State enacted the precedent-setting Poor House Act of 1824, which transferred responsibility for aid from the towns to the counties, states played a very limited role in public assistance. The local community would assume responsibility for the needy only if families were unable to do so. The major responsibility—financial, legal, and moral—rested with the family unit (Achenbaum, 1978). Many states passed legislation dealing explicitly with the issue of dependency and poverty. It is not known, however, whether states enacted laws requiring family members to be responsible for their poor or infirm kin "in order to preclude a possible failure of the family to care for its own poor or whether they were responding to actual changes in relatives' ability or willingness to assume such responsibility" (Achenbaum, 1978, p. 76). When families could not meet this obligation, the dependent individual had little choice but to seek shelter in a public almshouse.

Before the Civil War an estimated 25 percent of the resident population of public almshouses was over 60 years of age. State and local governments raised the funds to build these facilities without any particular concern for the aged. Those unfortunate enough to be old, poor, and without family got the same treatment as did criminals or vagrants. By the turn of the century, there was a rise in the proportion of destitute elderly residing in almshouses, and, in fact, some almshouses were converted into homes for the aged. In 1910, roughly 45 percent of the native-born and 70 percent of the foreign-born inmates of almshouses were at least 60 years of age (Achenbaum, 1978, p. 80). The private sector attempted to respond to the need of some older persons by establishing old age homes or "benevolent homes" as an alternative to the workhouse. In addition, many state legislatures dealt with the basic need for income support in old age by considering or enacting measures to provide pensions to certain categories of residents in their states, for example, veterans, firemen, and police (Achenbaum, 1978).

These early trends indicate that, although there was a general aversion to a U.S. welfare state, the role of the state was becoming increasingly important by default if not by design. These early state poor law measures demonstrated the shifting organization of support for older members from the family to a more collective social effort (Myles, 1984). The basic concept of *social* welfare was also a distinct move away from the social unit of family, individual, and parish to the larger social organization of the state. Welfare as a form of social insurance meant state intervention to protect the population against the risks of calamities due to illness or loss of employment and income. Formidable barriers against acceptance of this idea existed— not the least of which was the U.S. ideology of individualism and voluntarism in a classless society (Morison and Commager, 1962). This ideology suggested that each person had an equal chance to get rich in the United States, therefore, being poor or without property was attributable to one's own ignorance, folly, or sloth. The theory of Social Darwinism, immensely popular in the United States, legiti-mized these beliefs (Lubove, 1968). According to Achenbaum (1983), the evolution of federal programs and policies for the aged in America has been characterized by ambiguity and conflict arising from such value dichotomies as self-reliance/dependency, individual/family, private/public, equity/adequacy, and expectation/entitlement.

Two pervasive and enduring beliefs that have worked against the development of the U.S. welfare state for the aged are the belief that individuals create their own conditions and opportunities and thus have only themselves to blame for their predicament and the belief that the cost of government intervention is harmful to the productivity and economic well-being of the nation. Both of these beliefs emerged on the platform of public debate during the Depression. Now, fifty years later in the 1980s, the debate about the fiscal and moral responsibility for the nation's older citizens is based on these same beliefs (Estes and Gerard, 1983).

The Progressive Era

Following the end of the Civil War in 1865, there was a tremendous growth in industrialization and urbanization. By 1920 the United States had grown from its status as a secondary industrial nation in 1860 to a position of "industrial preeminence" (Jackson and Schultz, 1972, p. 177). This economic expansion was fueled by an unprecedented influx of immigrants and by the migration of workers from rural farm areas to the major industrial cities, which held the promise of a better life. It is not surprising, then, that the Progressive Era (1900–1920) is often characterized as a period of "social turmoil and intense competition among different social groupings and classes for political power and influence in the United States" (Weinstein, 1968, p. 3). One of the central concerns of the progressive reform movements at the turn of the century was to establish the right of workers to secure and maintain a decent standard of living and to strengthen the role of government in protecting that right (Rimlinger, 1971).

The force of industrialism in the United States created the socioeconomic conditions that necessitated a change in the limited role of government in social domestic affairs. The attitudes isolating illness to the private, personal sphere also began to change. Prior to the expansion of the industrial sector of the economy, illness was regarded simply as a private problem. This changed rather rapidly as industry leaders recognized the importance of an able-bodied, healthy work force. Once the wave of immigration had receded, control and reliability of labor became an issue to managers in the industrial, urban states. Industrialization helped move illness from the private sphere to the collective, social sphere. According to Starr (1982), the "demand for health insurance originated in the breakdown of a household economy as families came to depend on the labor of their chief wage earner for income and on the services of doctors and hospitals for medical treatment" (p. 236).

Up until the New Deal legislation, the dominant method of dealing with dependency resulting from poverty, sickness, or unemployment was through voluntary, private charity organizations and/or local government assistance guided by poor law legislation. This method favored institutional public assistance relief. Local governmental and private philanthropic discretion was used to determine need and prescribe a remedy. Voluntary charitable institutions, as well as the emerging field of social work, adopted a perspective largely unmindful of the objective causes of poverty and unemployment. They concentrated instead on the *subjective* causes of poverty—character, morality, deviance. The goals of such philanthropic endeavors were not only to provide economic relief for the destitute but also to serve as a means of socialization and education, inculcating such values as self-reliance, industriousness, the Protestant work ethic, and thrift (Lubove, 1968).

Organized political efforts to deal with the *objective* causes of dependency—poverty, illness, injury, unemployment, death of a spouse, and old age—are part of the archives of the larger story of class struggle between labor and capital (Lubove, 1968; Rimlinger, 1971; Myles, 1984). In 1906, the American Association for Labor Legislation (AALL) was established. By 1911, this organization had launched the social insurance movement in the United States (Lubove, 1968). As an organization, the AALL did not seek to mobilize mass support for the concept of social insurance but rather directed its efforts to employers, government and civic leaders, and intellectuals (Rimlinger, 1971). The membership of AALL consisted of social scientists in the areas of economics and political science, including Henry Farnam from Yale, J. W. Jenks from Cornell, Henry Seager and Samuel McCune Linsay from Columbia, John R. Commons and Richard Ely from Wisconsin, John B. Andrews, Isaac M. Rubinow, and A. F. Weber.

I. M. Rubinow, a noted American physician and major theoretician of social insurance, had a vision of the historical inevitability of social insurance, which he defined as the "policy of organized society to furnish that protection to one part of the population which some other part may need less, or needing, is able to purchase voluntarily through private insurance" (Lubove, 1968, p. 36). Rubinow recognized the wage-earner's dependence on the labor market and the vulnerability of the worker to such risks as injury, illness, or old age, any of which could interrupt the flow of earnings. Rubinow was convinced that social insurance was "a logical response to income maintenance problems inherent in a wage-centered, industrial economy" (Lubove, 1968, p. 36). The concept of social insurance, as articulated by Rubinow, differed significantly from the principles of private insurance or public assistance at that time. The introduction of such notions as compulsion, cost participation by employers and the state, and public insurance institutions were considered quite radical. According to Lubove:

> The social insurance movement was a thrust toward rationalization of the American welfare system; it aspired to centralization, the transfer of functions from the private to the public sector, and a new definition of the role of the government in American life. (1968, p. 3)

This movement for social insurance, in turn, gave rise to the earliest organized political efforts to establish compulsory health insurance, viewed by reformers as part of the right to income security. The major reform effort was concentrated on the health and safety of workers in such major industries as railroads, iron, and steel where industrial accidents sometimes resulted in injury or death (Lubove, 1968). In fact, the very first measure of social insurance enacted was workmen's compensation—insurance against the risk of temporary disability and/or loss of income. Second in priority was health insurance, followed by unemployment insurance. These priorities changed with the Depression of the 1930s, but at that time reformers anticipated health insurance would follow workmen's compensation. However, given the strength of political influence of doctors and insurance companies, the goal of compulsory health insurance was a highly controversial one. In the heat of the debate over social welfare policy and programs, then and now, the microeconomic ends of these programs often were overlooked.

A number of studies (Rimlinger, 1971; Lubove, 1968; Graebner, 1980; Skocpol and Ikenberry, 1982) have emphasized the importance of the political environment, played out most dramatically between organized labor and capital, and how this worked to shape progressive reforms during this period. Urban violence, racial conflict, militant labor, and massive industrial accidents set the stage for industry's new priorities—efficiency and control (Graebner, 1980). Although the industrialists' seat of power would not yield readily to union demands, some leaders in the private business sector foresaw how some of the concerns for income security might serve their needs. Graebner's (1980) study of U.S. retirement and social security legislation exemplifies how one form of social insurance, the old age pension, serves a variety of microeconomic institutional goals. In order to maximize profit and productivity, industrial capitalists needed to consider such factors as reducing turnover of personnel, maintaining and providing promotional opportunities, replacing inefficient older workers with younger ones and expensive salaried personnel with less expensive ones, and allowing employers to defer wage increases or to lower salaries through deferral of benefits (Graebner, 1980). The concept of superannuation (payments by employers to retired workers) became more acceptable to employers as they began to see an opportunity not only to control the labor supply but also to combat union organizing by offering small pensions as a token of concern. Old age pensions also served a symbolic function of showing a paternalistic face to the public during a period of extreme violence between industry and labor (Calhoun, 1978).

Similarly, the movement for compulsory health insurance for workers was organized by the AALL at least partially to serve other goals. Early reform efforts were tied to the goals of conservation and efficiency of human resources in order to appeal to the self-interest of industrial employers (Rimlinger, 1971). It is noteworthy that the older worker was not singled out or set apart during this stage of the movement for health insurance protection. However, it was recognized that older persons were made economically vulnerable by retirement and further by the possible onset of illness or disability.

The identification of different types of economic costs incurred by the onset of illness or disability is useful in understanding the origins of the struggle for health insurance. There are two general kinds of costs: (1) the indirect costs of the loss of income and wages to the individual and the loss of diminished productivity to industry, and (2) the direct costs of individual medical costs and costs to the state (Starr, 1982, p. 236). Table 3-1 shows the two types of costs. The movement for health insurance originally focused on the indirect costs—protecting the worker against loss of income due to illness or death. It was not until the 1930s that the movement shifted its focus to the direct costs, thereby ensuring wider public support from the middle- and upper-income classes (Starr, 1982).

Table 3-1
Types of Economic Costs Incurred by Illness or Disability

Indirect costs (capital and labor)	Direct costs (value of resources used to prevent or treat health problems)
Loss of income, that is, wages for individual or family in caretaker role	*Individual medical costs*, that is, private medical expenditures, insurance premiums
Loss of or diminished productivity output to industry, that is, absenteeism, necessity of replacement, impact on general productivity	*Costs to the state*, that is, medical care, tax revenues/public monies spent

Health insurance for workers was advocated in light of its appeal to industry for a more efficient, stable, and healthy work force (Rimlinger, 1971; Starr, 1982). The concept of health insurance was introduced as part of an overall strategy of income maintenance for wage earners to increase efficiency (that is, productivity), prevent disease, and relieve poverty (Starr, 1982). In economic terms, health insurance was advocated to industrial employers as an investment in "human capital." Progressive reform proposals introduced the concept of compulsory health insurance (a mixture of German and English systems) as a major benefit both to the worker in terms of the indirect costs of illness in the form of wage loss and to the employer in terms of the indirect costs of diminished productivity and loss of workers (Starr, 1982, p. 244).

The educational and political reform efforts of the AALL had a major effect. Health insurance became a key political topic of debate among labor unions, employers, civic leaders, and state legislators. The notion of protecting workers against the risks of illness was gaining both public and professional support. Leaders of the medical profession, who supported the AALL proposals, were involved in designing a model of health insurance (Starr, 1982). As the new decade of the 1920s approached, however, opposition, especially from physicians, the insurance industry, and employers, began to grow. In addition, the entry of the United States into World War I in 1917 had a major effect on the progressive movement, diminishing its capacity and diverting attention away from social reform.

The period following World War I was one of complacency in terms of the health insurance issue. It was, however, a period in which the aged emerged as a notable political force. Well before the onset of the Depression, the demand for old age protection was gaining political support. Rimlinger (1971) attributes this to two basic factors. First, demographic trends indicated that the U.S. population was aging, with a rise in the 65 and over age group from 2.7 percent of the population in 1860 to 5.4 percent in 1930, numerically more than doubling between 1900 and 1930. Second, the high cost of relief in poorhouses, which was the only alternative left to many needy older persons, increased the financial burden on society. Ironically, it was the institutional character of relief policy, or at least the economic factors of institutionalization, that urged public officials to reassess policy. The social insurance activists were superseded by leaders of some newly founded organizations, the American Association for Old Age Security, the Fraternal Order of Eagles, and the Townsend Club (Lubove, 1968; Pratt, 1976). A number of studies have documented this period of political struggle for income security in old age (Altmeyer, 1966; Douglas, 1936; Holtzman, 1963; Epstein, 1936;

Pratt, 1976), which laid the groundwork for the Social Security Act in 1935.

The New Deal, Social Security, and Health

It took the conditions of the Great Depression—a mass of unemployed persons and bankruptcies among large and small businesses—to dramatically change political opinion on the role and responsibilities of the federal government. Prior to this event, the dominant belief was that misfortune was the individual's own fault and that the responsibility for general welfare of citizens rested with charity, local government, or whatever self-help initiative the individual could exercise.

In the United States and other Western capitalist democracies, the practice of economic policy and the theory of political economy underwent major revisions. John Maynard Keynes's (1965) *General Theory of Employment, Interest, & Money* helped to redefine the economic responsibilities of the central government and conveyed a basic optimism about the compatibility of capitalism and social democracy (Tobin, 1981). In June of 1934, President Franklin D. Roosevelt addressed Congress concerning the federal role in the economic security of citizens:

> If, as our Constitution tells us, our federal government was established among other things, to promote the general welfare, it is our plain duty to provide for that security upon which welfare depends. (1938, p. 291)

One year later, the most significant piece of social legislation in U.S. history—the Social Security Act of 1935—was enacted and signed into law. This event marked the founding of the U.S. welfare state (Derthick, 1979). In addition to the compulsory federal old-age retirement program (Title II) and unemployment insurance (Title III), the act also included optional grants-in-aid to states for old age pensions based on need (Title I), aid to dependent children (Title IV), and maternal and child welfare services and rehabilitation for crippled children (Titles V and VI).

In terms of financing, coverage, and payments to unemployed and retired workers, the Social Security Act of 1935 was limited, especially when compared to European standards (Derthick, 1979). However, this legislation has been referred to as a watershed in U.S. history because it marked a turning point in thinking about domestic social needs. There was an unprecedented expansion of the federal role. However, the federal government moved cautiously so as to maintain a balance of power and authority in federal and state intergovernmental relations. The New Deal ushered in a new concept of federal-state relations known as cooperative federalism—a partnership between the federal and state governments (D. Walker, 1981). This partnership was basically a political compromise between the urgent need for national uniform policy in the area of individual economic security and the preservation of traditional state and local authority in other areas of defining needs and administering benefits to the poor.

Thus the Social Security Act represented an amalgam of philosophies that were to become the basis for future domestic social policy. The provisions of the act made a clear separation between the entitlement rights of workers who deserved income protection with national standards and of those outside of the labor market or in the secondary labor market. The latter groups had not earned their rights and were (and are) subject to the political will of states and localities or of voluntary private institutions of charity. As Rimlinger has noted:

> Although the American Social Security Act never formally recognized a status hierarchy among citizens, it left the door open to many inequalities of protection, especially as between the residents of different states. (1971, p. 224)

Old age pensions and unemployment insurance under the Social Security Act addressed the idea of a citizen's right to income security on a nationwide scale, without means-tested criteria. On the other hand, other parts of the act directly addressed the economic concerns of destitute and impoverished individuals and a state's fiscal capacity to meet these needs. For example, Title I of the Social Security Act of 1935, which was to become the basis for welfare assistance for almost forty years, provided broad discretion to the states in determining eligibility and the amount of payments; impoverished individuals still had to demonstrate need and be subjected to the social stigma associated with charity at the state and local levels of government.

In summary, from the inception of the Social Security Act, the dual concepts of social insurance benefits and welfare benefits have served to foster distinctively different types of health programs (Stevens and Stevens, 1974; Brown, 1982; Skocpol and Ikenberry, 1982).

Faith in the ideology of individualism and self-help was eroded in the United States by the direct experience of the Depression, and support for federal intervention was strong and widespread. Yet a salient aspect of coverage excluded from the Social Security Act of 1935 (particularly in light of the preceding twenty years of reform efforts) was health insurance. Starr (1982) contends that health was excluded from the New Deal package not because of the lack of public support but because of the political and economic power of physicians and insurance companies, who defeated legislation that would infringe on their professional sovereignty and profit.

The issue of health, although excluded from the Social Security Act of 1935, still remained an important unresolved national problem. Under presidential initiative, the Technical Committee on Medical Care was established in 1937 to review the health problem and make recommendations. This committee, like the previous Committee on Economic Security, emphasized federal subsidies to the states to "operate health programs instead of a national health insurance system" (Starr, 1982, p. 276). The committee's recommendations included proposals (1) to expand public health and maternal and child health services under the Social Security Act, (2) to expand hospital facilities and aid for medical care for welfare recipients in the form of federal aid to the states, and (3) to initiate federal action toward a program of compensation for wage losses due to temporary or permanent disability (Starr, 1982, p. 276).

National health insurance was divested of its original fervor and reexamined in light of professional and corporate interests and in light of a welfare tradition that stratified health care and separated the poor from the middle and upper classes. The need for health protection for the working and retired populations was postponed at least until after World War II when, again, it was to emerge with a new political face.

The Evolution of Separate Systems: Medicare and Medicaid

No other country in the world, observes Marmor (1970), began its government health program with the aged. Yet in the United States this was exactly where the political debate for health insurance focused after World War II. Under the leadership of organized labor, a national health plan for all workers was advocated and sought (Marmor, 1970; Munts, 1967; Falk, 1964). The post–World War II climate, however, was hardly favorable to such proposals. Opponents of national health insurance were able to utilize anti-German and anticommunist sentiments to undermine national health proposals and to polarize the nation around the heated issue of socialism versus capitalism (Starr, 1982).

Conflicts among health advocates, labor activists, the American Medical Association, the insurance industry, and political party leaders were long and often bitter. Events surrounding and shaping "the long war" (Harris, 1969) leading up to the final passage of Medicare in 1965 are contained in works providing detailed accounts of the dramatic play of power (Harris, 1969; Marmor, 1970; Rose, 1967; Law, 1974; Feder, 1977). The focus of our attention is on the enduring conflict of values and the human and political consequences for health care for the aged. The post–World War II debate included issues of compulsory versus voluntary insurance and citizen entitlement rights versus charity, or means-tested relief programs. Each of these dichotomies involved political choices concerning the individual and the nation state, and the national-state-local division of responsibility and authority. Although carried over from the earlier progressive movement for social insurance, these concepts continued to be salient political issues in the debate over health insurance. These issues emerged during the 1950s and had a decisive impact on shaping the legislation of the 1960s. In effect, these issues solidified a distinctly stratified system of health care for older persons.

The Republicans' plan for the nation's health was to strictly separate compulsory and voluntary health insurance along class lines. During the Truman Administration (about 1946–49), the Republicans emphasized "a system of welfare medicine for the poor financed by federal aid and administered by the participating states" (Starr, 1982, p. 284). In responding to criticism that such a plan would segregate the poor from other citizens and subject them to the social stigma of means-tested charity, Senator Robert Taft retorted that compulsory health insurance should be the medicine for the poor and they should "have to take it the way the State says to take it" (Starr, 1982, p. 284). Fearing that a universal approach would lower the demand for their services, physicians also argued for means-tested health insurance (Harris, 1969). The means test

> was at the heart of the ensuing controversy. A program that provided medical care only for those who were unable to pay for it at the market price made that care charity. On the other hand, a program that provided medical care for Social Security beneficiaries under an insurance system that they had contributed to made that care an earned right. (Harris, 1969, p. 61)

By the 1950s, labor's objective had shifted from national health insurance to an insurance mechanism for retired workers and their dependents. Numerous bills were introduced in Congress throughout the 1950s to provide health care for the aged (Rimlinger, 1971). Late in 1956, the AFL-CIO renewed the movement for some form of health insurance for the elderly. Nelson Cruickshank, Robert Ball, Wilbur Cohen, and I. S. Falk were the first architects of a "new and greatly expanded bill to provide medical care for social security beneficiaries" (Harris, 1969, p. 72). Following a protracted ideological and economic struggle between industry and organized labor over the question of health insurance, another shift in strategy was undertaken. By the early 1960s, the National Coalition of Senior Citizens (NCSC) was established as the major lobbyist and advocate for health protection for the aged (Rose, 1967; Marmor, 1970). Between 1961 and 1965, the three largest economic interest groups in health, the hospitals, physicians, and insurance industry, took a dominant role in shaping the insurance plan (later known as Medicare) (Marmor, 1970; Rose, 1967; Law, 1974). Finally, in the summer of 1965, the Medicare program was enacted (Title XVIII of the Social Security Act)—"making the United States the last industrialized nation in the West to adopt a compulsory health insurance program" (Harris, 1969, p. 3).

This background to the passage of public health insurance merely outlines the involved and complex network of interaction among key actors, vested economic interests, and the federal government. Several important facets of the historical development of health protection for the aged emerge.

1. Medicare was designed as a Social Security improvement, not a medical care reform measure. In fact, the Medicare law "explicitly promised that the federal insurance program would not interfere in the practice of medicine or the structure of the medical care industry" (Feder, 1977, p. 174).
2. Medicare was a very specific piece of legislation to redress the problem created by retirement policies that, in effect, reduced the individual's ability to meet the direct costs of illness.
3. Medicare was a shift to the direct economic costs incurred by receipt of medical care bills. Medicare was to underwrite a large share of the costs of inpatient hospital care and physician services associated with episodes and treatment of acute illness.
4. The long unresolved conflict between private and public interests was settled by dividing the program in two parts: only the hospital insurance (Part A) was made compulsory and prepaid through social insurance; physician and other outpatient services (Part B) were put on a voluntary but federally subsidized basis (Rimlinger, 1971).
5. Medicare established an entitlement program to health insurance based on age. Legitimacy surrounding the program arose out of the very framework of the program as an entitlement earned from

labor market participation; this is reflected in the financing by payroll tax on employer and employee.

This distinctly American attitude of getting what you paid for—at least in theory, if not in practice—imbued the Medicare program with the idea that health care for retired workers was a matter of "earned right" (Harris, 1969; Marmor, 1970). This important and hard won concept unfortunately did not extend to everyone in need. The segment of the population that did not meet the age or disability criteria of Medicare but was unable to pay for the cost of illness was relegated to a separate system of welfare medicine (Stevens and Stevens, 1974). This separate and unequal system of welfare medicine often meant individuals were subject to the high stigma associated with poverty and means-tested charity programs run by state and local governments. The more generous view of medical need assigned a deserving status to mothers and children and blind or aged recipients of public assistance because it was thought that their dependency was, at least, a temporary or unalterable condition of nature.

Even though the Social Security legislation was the basis for both Medicare and Medicaid, the two programs diverged radically in concept, certainty, stigma, coverage, and determination of need and benefits. Table 3-2 outlines the incremental steps in the development of health insurance for the poor from 1935 until the passage of Medicaid in 1965. The Social Security Act of 1935 included a provision for a very minimal amount of payment to states for medical expenses incurred by welfare recipients. Prior to this, the cost for the provision of medical care assistance for the poor was left entirely to the states and localities. However, there was no significant federal action in health care for the poor (Holahan, 1975) until the 1950 amendments to the Social Security Act. These amendments provided for federal matching funds to the states for payment of medical services directly to physicians, hospitals, and other providers.

Legislative opponents of health insurance adopted strategies of delay and preemption. It was in this political context that the Kerr-Mills Act was adopted in 1960 (Derthick, 1979). The federal role was enlarged to a greater extent by the passage of this act (amendment to Title I of the Social Security Act). In addition to providing federal matching grants to states for the provision of medical care to a state's welfare population, the 1960 amendment authorized medical assistance for the aged, the first public assistance program aimed at assisting near-poor, "medically needy" individuals who were unable to cover the cost of medical care. The Kerr-Mills Act of 1960 was important as a first step in public financing of health care for America's elderly citizens, many of whom were living at the near-poor income level. This legislation was, however, limited. Eligibility for public financing of health care for the aged was closely linked to state

Table 3-2
Incremental Steps in Health Insurance for the Poor

Year	Step
1935	Passage of the Social Security Act of 1935 (P.L. 74–271) included federal matching of payments for medical expenses incurred by welfare recipients. States' participation was optional. The act expanded the federal role by offering the states funds on a matching basis for maternal and infant care, care for children under age 16, rehabilitation of crippled children, and general public health measures.
1950	Federal matching funds were made available to the states for vendor payments of physicians, hospitals, and other providers of medical care for those on public assistance (the poorest).
1960	The Kerr-Mills Amendment increased the federal financial role by providing higher levels of federal matching grants under Title I Old Age Assistance. It created a new category, medical assistance for the aged, for those who proved financial need for assistance with medical bills. Participation by the states was optional. Use of assistance varied greatly as each state set its own standard of medical and financial need.
1965	Medicaid (Title XIX of the Social Security Act) enacted. This legislation continued the basic welfare approach to medical assistance for the poor, increased federal financial participation, and mandated minimum coverage to a state's welfare population.

welfare structure, policy, and ideology. Benefits were provided only to the most needy, and benefits varied considerably from state to state.

Federal leadership in ensuring access to services and an equitable distribution of benefits across states was virtually nonexistent. As Stevens commented, "Kerr-Mills was perhaps less a means of increasing aid to the elderly than it was a means for shifting the burden of that aid from others to the federal government" (p. 30). The most distinguishing feature of this legislation was that it was "predicated on a welfare, means-oriented not a social security insurance theory" (Stevens and Stevens, 1974, p. 31).

The advent of the Medicare program spurred state governments to lobby Congress for increased federal participation in health care for the poor. The Medicaid program was passed in 1965 largely as a concession to the states, which had argued that the federal government should expand its share of the financing of medical assistance for the poor. Medicaid's primary aim was "not to provide health care as a right to needy groups but to provide services only to the extent that medical bills would not defeat the purpose of programs for income assistance" (Stevens and Stevens, 1974, p. 319).

The 1965 Medicaid legislation continued the basic welfare approach to medical assistance for the poor, which still underlies the structure of Medicaid eligibility today (Davidson and Marmor, 1980). The major differences of the 1965 legislation were the unification of the categorical grants under one single program, the increased rate of federal financial participation in the costs of medical care, and the mandates concerning coverage of a state's welfare population and the types of services to be provided. States were also encouraged to include the medically needy, those persons who were near poor and could not afford to meet the costs of medical care, in their Medicaid program (Holahan, 1975).

In summary, Medicaid is distinguished from Medicare in several important ways. First, it was designed as a welfare program, and as such has stigmatized the poor with means-tested eligibility. Second, it presented an incentive to state governments in that it was to be a shared federal-state financial responsibility for medical care of the poor. Medicaid, unlike Medicare, is a joint federal and state program. The federal match, ranging from 50 to 78 percent, has assisted states in financing the cost of provision of health services. At the same time states have been allowed broad discretion in administration and determination of eligibility and scope of services. Third, Medicaid evolved out of the social conditions of the Depression and emphasized health care as a market commodity to be purchased for the poor by third-party payers. One of the stated purposes of the Medicaid program was to provide the poor with access to mainstream medicine by direct reimbursement to private physicians and other health care providers. It would appear that the aged who were indigent fell into the welfare medicine stigma rather by default than by design.

Overview

The differences between public welfare (Medicaid) and social insurance (Medicare) are summarized in Table 3-3, which presents a comparative chart of the five systems of health care for older persons. Although not directly applicable to the provision of services, federal tax policy must be included in the stratified system of care as an important indirect source of financing for upper-income groups (Wilensky, 1982; Nelson, 1983). Unlike other public programs resulting in direct federal expenditures, tax provisions in the form of medical deductions and the exclusion of employer contributions for medical insurance premiums and medical care are indirect federal expenditures amounting to over $21 billion in 1983 (U.S. Congress, Joint Committee on Taxation, 1983).

Private insurance has been an important supplement to Medicare; at least 16 million elderly persons purchased some form of coverage from private industry in 1979 (Long, Settle, and Link, 1982). Medicare's share of all personal health expenditures for the elderly accounts for about 45 percent. The gaps in service coverage (for example, physician services, drugs, eyeglasses, podiatry, dental work, and hearing care) must be paid out of pocket or by private insurance. Although millions hold private insurance policies, actual coverage is so limited as to be almost inconsequential, paying for less than 6 percent of the health expenditures for the elderly (Ball, 1981).

Veterans' health care is the oldest publicly funded system in the United States. It has evolved since 1811 into what is now the "largest centrally coordinated health care system in the nation" (U.S. Senate, 1977b, p. 204) with outlays of $8.9 billion for hospital, medical care, and construction (U.S. House, 1983). Although originally designed as an acute care system for veterans, the Veterans Administration has developed a wide spectrum of health care services, including hospitals, nursing homes, outpatient clinics, and domiciliary homes. In addition, contracts are made with the nonfederal sector for services. This system of care is an important source of non–means-tested, prepaid health care for older men. It is anticipated that the aging of the veteran population will increase the demand for both acute and long-term care in the next twenty years. It is projected that more than one-fourth of the veterans (7.1 million) will be over 64 years of age by the year 2000 (U.S. Senate, 1977a). Health costs for veterans, unlike other public programs, have always held the distinction of being what George Washington referred to as "a debt of honor" (U.S. Senate, 1977b, p. 202). Medical care was provided only for service-connected disabilities until 1924, when hospitalization coverage was extended to all veterans without regard to the nature or origin of their disabilities. Access to care, however, varies by region and type of service needed, with the main priority given to those with service-connected disabilities.

It should be emphasized that these systems are not exclusive of each other; they often intersect in some important ways, depending on health, age, and employment status. For example, private insurance is available to the majority of workers in the U.S. labor force under some type of group health plan in their place of employment. Coverage varies according to industry, length of employment, and geographic location but is generally extended to the families of these workers also. However, as a result of high levels of unemployment in the United States in the past several years, many workers and their families—the Congressional Budget Office estimates over 10 mil-

Table 3-3
Stratified Systems in the Provision and Financing of Health Care
for Older Persons

	Social insurance (Medicare)	Public welfare (Medicaid)
Benefit concept	"Earned" right derived from labor market	Charity, derived from welfare principle
Financing	Payroll taxes and general revenue	General revenue (federal) and state/local government taxes
Criteria	Age and disability factors (65 years plus)	Means-tested, pauperization (mainly aged, blind, disabled, children, and mothers)
Stigma	None, social insurance	Very high, charity
Coverage	Universal (Part A compulsory; Part B voluntary)	Highly variable, determined by welfare policies
Certainty	High, subject to national commitment and economic growth	None, vulnerable to swings in state level capacity and political commitment
Access to service	High, hospital services tied to ability to pay deductibles and copayments and willingness of providers to participate	Variable, tied to availability of supply and willingness of providers to serve the poor and ability to pay cost sharing in some states

lion—have lost their employment-based group health benefits and their employers' contributions toward the costs of health protection (U.S. Senate, 1983). Older workers are particularly hard hit during times of recession. Persons 55 years of age and over experience a much higher rate of unemployment than do younger persons (U.S. House, Select Committee on Aging, 1982). For many older persons, this may mean forced early retirement and living with fewer financial resources because of the difficulty of getting another job. Having lost the ability to pay, the major criterion for entry into the private health care system, millions of people have been forced to forgo adequate and even minimal protection against the risk of illness. A small percentage of the unemployed may be eligible for state-administered

Tax laws	Private insurance	Veterans' benefits
Expenses and earnings derived from fiscal policy	Class privilege derived from the market	Earned by military service
Indirect federal spending	Individual, group, or employer	General revenue
Deductibility of medical expenses above a percentage of adjusted income	Ability to pay	Veteran of active duty with honorable discharge
None, IRS entitlement	None, highly approved	None, "debt of honor"
Not applicable	Carrier discretion or negotiated	Universal
High, national fiscal policy	High, subject to health status, sex, age factors	High, governed by statutory eligibility requirements
Not applicable	Assured but relative burden of cost sharing and premium payment rises as income falls	High for service-connected conditions

programs, but strict eligibility requirements in most states preclude access for most. A select number who served on active duty in the armed services may be able to seek care for themselves through the veterans' system of health care (U.S. Senate, 1983).

In summary, there really is no single national, comprehensive health insurance for the aged. Medicare insures retired workers against the risks of large, institutional (and often catastrophic) medical care costs, and Medicaid insures the poorest population, those deemed state-welfare eligibles, against the costs of medical care. Both programs are not so much systems of care as financing mechanisms to meet medical vendor payments for services contracted from the private and public sectors.

Chapter

4

The Medical-Industrial Complex

People in the United States are now spending $280 billion per year, nearly 10 percent of the gross national product, on health, which is a larger commitment to health than is made by any other nation (Ricardo-Campbell, 1982). Relative to the U.S. economy in general, the health care industry has grown rapidly, and health care is now among the top five "industries" in the United States (Gibson and Waldo, 1981). Rising costs of health care have been a major concern at all levels of government (Gibson and Waldo, 1982; Davis, 1982). The growth of health care expenditures has been attributed to health care price inflation (as much as 60–75 percent), population increases (about 8 percent) and intensity of care (about 28 percent) in the use of technology, equipment, and lab services. The past 15 years have been marked by medical care price inflation that has been considerably higher than the general rate of inflation. A "basket" of medical goods and services "that would have cost $100 in 1965 would have cost $329 in 1981" (Gibson and Waldo, 1982, p. 5). Table 4-1 shows national health expenditures for all ages and compares the rise in total dollars spent and per capita dollars for the years 1965, 1978, and 1982.

The sources of funding for health care for all age groups have changed markedly since the enactment of Medicare and Medicaid in 1965. These shifts are most dramatically evidenced in the financing of health care for the elderly. First, there has been a major shift in the proportion of the costs of this health care that is borne by the private and public sectors, as can be seen in comparisons over a short thirteen-year span. In 1965, the private sector paid 70 percent of the costs of personal health care for those 65 years of age and over, while the public sector paid 30 percent of the costs. By 1978, this share had

Table 4-1
National Health Expenditures (for all ages)

	1965	1978	1982
Total			
amount (billions of dollars)	41.7	189.3	322.4
per capita (dollars)	210.89	835.57	1365.0
percent of gross national product	6.0	8.8	10.5
Private sources			
amount (billions of dollars)	30.9	110.0	185.6
per capita (dollars)	156.32	485.29	786.0
percent of total	74.1	58.1	57.6
Public sources			
amount (billions of dollars)	10.8	79.4	136.8
per capita (dollars)	54.57	320.27	597.0
percent of total	25.9	41.9	42.4

Source: Gibson and Waldo, 1981 and 1982; Gibson, Waldo, and Levit, 1983.

nearly reversed itself, with the private sector assuming 36.8 percent of the cost and the public sector assuming 63.2 percent (Fisher, 1980). Second, there has been a shift in the levels of government financing health care for the elderly. In 1965, nearly half of the $2.6 billion of public funds expended on health care for persons 65 and older was from state and local governments. By 1978, the state-local government share was about one-seventh (or 14 percent) of the total $31 billion in public funds expended on health care for the elderly (Fisher, 1980). Nevertheless, in absolute dollars, even when adjusted for inflation, the states' burden of health costs has increased dramatically, due to the costs of Medicaid's long-term nursing care.

The provision and financing of medical care for the nation's older citizens has become a singularly important issue of public debate

Table 4-2
Distribution of Funding for Personal Health Care (age 65 years and over)

	1965	1978
Private	70.1%	36.8%
Public	29.9%	63.2%

Source: Fisher, C. R., 1980, p. 74, Table 6.

because the costs are so significant for both the state and federal levels. Health care for those over 65 years of age now absorbs about half of all public spending for personal health care (Fisher, 1980). Accelerated growth in hospital costs has resulted in substantial increases in the public share of expenditures for health. For every 1 percent increase in total hospital costs, federal outlays have increased by roughly $300 million (U.S. House, Committee on Ways and Means, 1982).

On a per capita basis, the $2,507 in health care expenditures for each older person is almost three times that for each of the other age groups. Although spending has been high, these benefits have been heavily concentrated among a small population. For example, in the Medicare program, only 12 percent of beneficiaries received benefits of over $2,000 per year, while the majority (77 percent) received benefits of $500 or less (Davis, 1982).

In 1981, expenditures for hospital care totaled $118 billion, with over half financed by public funds; nursing home expenditures totaled $24 billion, also with over half financed by public funds. Physician services totaled $54.8 billion, with over a quarter financed by public funds. Drug expenditures totaled $21.4 billion, largely financed by direct out-of-pocket payments. The two major sources of public health care funding for the elderly, Medicare and Medicaid, together paid out a total of $73 billion in benefits in 1981 (Gibson and Waldo, 1982). Figure 4-1 shows the percentage distribution of these two programs' funds for the different types of services. While hospital care services consumed the majority of funds under Medicare, nursing home care consumed the majority of funds under Medicaid.

Although federal contributions account for almost half of the nationwide Medicaid expenditures, this program has become a dominant factor in state health service provision and budgeting. Medicaid presently accounts for about one-third of state and local government health care expenditures (U.S. Congressional Budget Office, 1981b). Often it is the largest program in a state's budget (Freeland and Schendler, 1981). Since 1975, the role of Medicaid has become increasingly problematic because state fiscal capacity has not kept pace with program growth rate. Medicaid increases in expenditure have been one-third to one-half higher than the growth rates of state revenues (Bovbjerg and Holahan, 1982).

Changing Forces in U.S. Health Care

At numerous junctures in the development of the health industry, efforts have been made to realize a more rationalized health system,

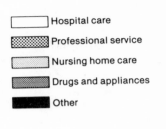

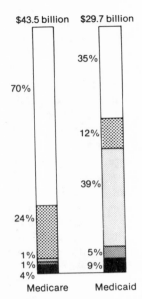

Figure 4-1. Personal Health Care Expenditures for Medicare and Medicaid: 1982

Source: Gibson, R. M., Waldo, D. R., and Levit, K. R., "National Health Expenditures, 1982." *Health Care Financing Review*, 5, No. 1 (Fall, 1983), pp. 1–31.

"one in which the parts are more coordinated hierarchically and horizontally and in which more emphasis is given to capital-intensive services" (Brown, 1979, p. 6). Brown (1979) traced back to the late 1920s to find the first efforts to rationalize medical care—the establishment of the General Education Board. This foundation was committed to shaping medical education to meet the standards of scientific and technological medicine. Brown summarized the impact such goals had on the organization of medical practice:

Private practice medicine had been founded upon simple, or petty, commodities that the physician himself could produce and sell. But technological medicine made physicians dependent on capital-intensive commodities, ones that require substantial capital investments and a good deal of hired labor to produce. For decades, this development redounded to the advantage of the profession. Medical technology enabled the profession and these new interest groups to further divide medical care into discrete service units and products that could be sold in the medical market. This intensive "commodification" of medical care enlarged the number of medical commodities that could be marketed. (1979, p. 198)

Financing for the scientific and technological aspects of medicine depended primarily on private foundations and wealthy donors. It was not until after World War II that the federal government played any significant role. The Hill-Burton Act of 1946 (Hospital Survey and Construction Act) was the first major subsidy to the private sector for expansion and construction of hospitals.

Efforts to rationalize the system clearly did not resolve such problems as high and uncontrollable costs, inequality of access to service, or fragmentation. However, the emerging forces of scientific knowledge, technical expertise and technologic innovation did indeed present a major challenge to the physician monopoly of health care (Stewart, 1968; Kelman, 1971). Kelman (1971) has theorized that the primary contradiction in the development of the U.S. medical care system was the incompatibility of technology in medicine with the private fee-for-service practice and the control of medicine traditionally exercised by the American Medical Association. In Kelman's analysis (1971), the reasons for this are that the introduction of science and technology necessitated an industrial base (that is, hospital expansion) and also required a substantial financing base for the delivery of medical care (that is, insurance companies and their associates in the banking industry). Thus, while the material conditions of advanced scientific knowledge and technology created the groundwork for change, the insurance companies and banks emerged as the key political forces in the industrialization of health (Kelman, 1971).

However, the federal government has been equally important in the industrialization of health. Since World War II, the federal role has expanded as Congress passed legislation and authorized money for research, education, training, and financing of health services. The passage of Medicare and Medicaid in 1965 played a pivotal part in the expansion of the medical-industrial complex. These programs expanded the federal role as third-party payer for health care services. The transformation from medical needs to public demand for health was secured. The Medicare and Medicaid programs served as an important source of long-term capital financing for hospitals. National expenditures for hospital care went from $13.9 billion in 1965 to $27.8 billion in 1970 to $135.5 billion in 1982 (Gibson, Waldo, and Levit, 1983). Overall, federal financing of health care performs the very important functions of sustaining aggregate demand through health insurance programs, protecting against financial risks, subsidizing research and guaranteeing substantial financial returns, supporting the system's infrastructure through training subsidies and capital expansion, and regulating competition through licensure and accreditation (LeRoy, 1979).

In diagnosing the malady of the health care system at the beginning of the 1970s, analysts both inside and outside of government agreed that the United States had a wasteful "nonsystem"—a cottage industry dominated by small, inefficient, and uncoordinated enterprises (Stewart, 1968; Ehrenreich and Ehrenreich, 1971; Finch and Egeberg, 1969). Evidence of the "nonsystem" of health care in the United States included such problems as fragmentation of services, maldistribution of personnel and facilities, uncontrollable costs, and inequality of access to medical services for different population groups.

The rapid and dynamic push for change in health care over the past two decades has been attributed to the unique fusion of public commitment to health and the impact of technology. Stewart (1968) emphasized that

> this technological revolution challenges the fundamental basis of the non-system in health services [because] . . . in common with all our other exploding technologies, medical technology depends upon a system. It demands specialization and subspecialization. It requires effective interlocks . . . [and] complex and costly equipment which in turn demands complex and costly housing. (p. 17)

Specialized technology requires heavy capital investment and an expansion of the industrial base to house the equipment and personnel.

By the 1970s, the health service industry had undergone a fundamental shift as it "moved from the era of the 'cottage industry' to that of space exploration" (Kissick, 1973, p. 262). As one of the two most rapidly growing segments of the service economy in the 1970s, the health industry had increased in number of workers to approximately seven million by 1980. Hoos (1972) has referred to the labor changes of the 1970s as a case of "technological transfer." Highly skilled labor and scientific expertise has been deployed from the military-aerospace industry to the health care industry. This shift in the work force has paralleled the increased federal share for health care for the nation's poor and aged.

The Health Care Industry and the Competitive Model

The goals of the health service industry are not only to improve the health status of the population and to protect a plurality of vested interests but also, and more importantly, to strengthen and preserve the private sector in different ways. The health care industry functions economically in society as a source of growth, accumulation of profit, investment opportunity, and employment. It also maintains the "human capital"—the health of the able-bodied work force (Rodberg and Stevenson, 1977). It may not, however, do so in the most efficient, that is, profit-maximizing, way (Emrich, 1980).

The assertion that major parts of the health care industry are not maximizing profits merits a closer look. Emrich (1980) named two different approaches to the financing of hospitals: public investment and private autonomy. The latter is concerned with "the capacity to generate sufficient revenue to recover the full economic cost of providing service" (Emrich, 1980, p. 1) and thus with profit maximization. By contrast, a public investment approach takes the view that "the cost of debt capital is low and the prevailing perception of the cost of equity capital is that its cost is also low if not free" (Emrich, 1980, p. 11). This results in investment decisions, and decisions to offer services, that "ignore the role of profit entirely or relegate it to the role of merely one element in the decision process" (Emrich, 1980, p. 12). Investment capital may be seen as being low in cost or free when it is available through cost-based reimbursement, government grants, and donations. Thus, certain government (and some private sector) policies draw funds into the health industry in ways that are inefficient or irrational from the point of view of capitalist profit-maximizing logic.

Buchanan (1982) presented evidence that, in terms of net profits and internally generated funds, hospital and nursing home chains lag behind most other industries. At the same time, they are among the leaders in the ratio of capital expenditures to internally generated funds, and in terms of debt to equity. Buchanan (1982, p. 313) referred to this sector of the health industry as a "cash guzzler constantly in need of outside funds." As shown in Figure 4-1, hospitals and nursing homes (along with physicians) are the major direct health providers to the aged. Because of the magnitude of their costs, the hospital and nursing home industries are of particular importance. These industries most directly link the health care industry to the larger economy.

That the hospital and nursing home industries are not on the whole as profitable as other private enterprises, that they have heavy capital expenditures financed largely by debt, and that they are not driven entirely by profit maximization do not, in and of themselves, bode ill for these industries. Hospitals and nursing homes provide a public good, and as a consequence, public policy has tended to subsidize or otherwise benefit them. However, given the magnitude of capital being absorbed by the health care industry and the rate of increase in the amount, it is unlikely that the hospital and nursing home industries will be allowed to continue as they have in the past. Insofar as its products are justified as a public good, the health care industry will continue to compete with other social expenditures in the face of economic and fiscal limits. Medicaid, for example, is seen by both federal and state governments as a large program with a potential for (or actuality of) expensive explosive growth resulting in a major drain on government resources.

On the other hand, insofar as sectors of the health care industry are justified on the basis of being part of a private sector industry, they will be judged by the same logic of profit maximization applied to other private sector industries. The rest of capital cannot look kindly on industries that have low profits, that heavily reinvest in themselves without consideration of alternatives, that rely heavily on debt financing (and are highly leveraged in terms of debt to equity), and that are major, rapidly growing industries. If the health care industries find debt financing to be cheap, their use of it will make debt financing more expensive for other industries competing for the same funds. If the practices of health care industries are subsidized or reimbursed by public funds derived from taxation, costs will be increased through higher taxation to other industries and to the economy as a whole. In short, it is quite likely that both public and private decision makers will attempt to "rein in" the hospital and nursing home industries, given the economic and fiscal crises and the rapid growth of these industries.

The concern about the profitability and efficiency of the health care industry has, in fact, been shared by policy makers. Major public policy shifts being introduced include the restructuring of the health care industry, the introduction of competition and the market into the industry, and the reform of government program reimbursement systems. Although it is not clear which of the many proposals now pending may ultimately be enacted, elements of these plans include:

· the raising of copayments and deductibles, and the use of voucher systems for public health care reimbursement to simulate "market choices" by consumers
· the encouragement, subsidy, or mandating of alternate health care provider structures such as HMO's, group practices, insurance company–sponsored health care groups, and hospital-based health systems
· the use of prospective payment contracting systems for public reimbursement programs
· the authorization for third-party insurers of prospective payment contracting with providers

· the taxation of employer contributions to employee health care plans, and full taxation of consumer medical expenses
· the encouragement of for-profit health care enterprises.

These initiatives involve (but do not all share) the following assumptions about the health care industry:

1. High costs are caused by health care choices by consumers.
2. Market mechanisms will ensure the most efficient and well-informed choices by consumers, as well as the quality of the product.
3. Health care services will be provided most efficiently by for-profit firms.
4. Government programs can ensure (a) adequate quality of care, with a minimum amount of regulation of providers, (b) reasonable reimbursement through prospective contracting with providers, and (c) an adequate health care "safety net" through simplified, perhaps federalized, insurance schemes or voucher systems.

Government Policy and the Medical-Industrial Complex

The market perspective dominating current health policy debate holds pluralism and fragmentation to be not only characteristic of the capitalist system but even healthy in guaranteeing diversity and in maintaining competition. Indeed, there is no doubt that pluralism, "the division of position, power, responsibility or obligation among groups or institutions" (Hiestand, 1971, p. 10), accurately typifies health care services in the United States; they are unique "in the pervasiveness of pluralism with respect to production, financing, and manpower" (Hiestand, 1971, p. 11). The commitment to a pluralistic, free market system is clearly shown in a health policy white paper developed in the 1970s by the Nixon Administration:

> Preference for action in the private sector is based on the fundamentals of our political economy—capitalistic, pluralistic, and competitive—as well as upon the desire to strengthen the capacity of our private institutions in their efforts to provide health services, to finance such services, and to provide the resources . . . . (U.S. Department of Health, Education, and Welfare, 1971, p. i)

Pluralism in health care may be a source of pride for those who stand to gain by the marketing of health products, or a source of confusion for those who are seeking or providing it. More importantly, pluralism in health raises some important questions about power and control over the production and distribution of health care resources.

In analyzing the exercise of the government's political and fiscal power to improve productivity and profitability in the private sector, especially the monopoly sector, O'Connor (1973) predicted that the United States may be moving toward a full scale social-industrial complex. He further argued that the "success of the social-industrial complex depends not only on strengthening the combined power of the state and monopoly capital, but also on weakening competitive capital, particularly its influence and power in local and state government and in Congress" (p. 56). Whether or not his prediction comes true remains to be seen, but there are an increasing number of examples of corporate management and control in health and human services, especially in halfway houses for adolescents and adults, hospitals, nursing homes, and home care. O'Connor's prediction of a social-industrial complex suggests that the "aging problem" and solutions to it may also succumb to the strict and calculating eye of market enthusiasts who wish to turn what society defines as "social junk" (for example, the aged) into private profit (Scull, 1977).

Beginning in the mid-1950s and continuing through the 1970s, the market for aging services and products expanded rapidly in the areas of housing, food, leisure, travel, and health (Calhoun, 1978). Much emphasis was placed on developing social services to meet the aged's new dependency and to reconstruct meaningful social roles for retired persons. The most lucrative market, however, was in health services, and this is the area which has expanded most rapidly.

Over ten years ago, the Ehrenreichs (1971) analyzed the U.S. health care system, arguing that improved health was not the only, or major, objective of this system. They delineated three functions of the U.S. health empire—profit-making, research, and education—and called attention to the "new medical-industrial complex." Drug manufacturers, suppliers of hospital materials and equipment, health insurance companies, hospitals, and nursing homes comprised the new medical-industrial complex and were among the major beneficiaries of the expanding public subsidy of health care. Table 4-3 highlights the composition of the American health empire in terms of national expenditures for selected services, research, and hospital construction activities in 1969 and 1982. Within a rather short period of time, a number of transformations have occurred in the medical-industrial complex in terms of the ownership and control of institutional structures. Starr commented on this change:

> In its original sense, the medical-industrial complex referred to the linkages between the doctors, hospitals, and medical schools and the health insurance companies, drug manufacturers, medical equipment

Table 4-3
U.S. Health Empire: Comparison of National Expenditures for
Years 1969 and 1982 (amounts in billions of dollars)

	1969	1982
Total national spending	$65.6	$322.4
Hospitals	24.1	135.5
Physicians	12.6	61.8
Drugs and medical sundries	7.1	22.4
Nursing homes	3.8	27.3
Research	1.9	5.9
Construction	2.9	8.2
Private share	62%	57.6%
Public share	38%	42.4%

Source: Gibson, R. M., Waldo, D. R., and Levit, K. R. "National Health Expenditures, 1982." *Health Care Financing Review*, 5, No. 1 (Fall, 1983), 1–31.

suppliers, and other profit-making firms. This early usage emphasized the hidden connections between industry and a medical system that was still made up almost entirely of independent practitioners and local, non-profit institutions. As of the early seventies, profit-making hospital and nursing home chains were visibly on the rise but still marginal to the health care system as a whole. (1982, pp. 428–429).

Relman (1980) has observed more recent developments of the medical-industrial complex that challenge the physician's monopoly on the way in which health care is paid for and provided. The new medical-industrial complex outlined by Relman is composed of four major sectors:

1. *Proprietary hospitals*, especially in the sunbelt states in the South, the Southwest, and along the Pacific coast, and outside the United States in underdeveloped countries as well as industrialized Western nations. These hospitals generate billions of dollars in profits.
2. *Proprietary nursing homes*, a multibillion dollar industry largely supported by public funds.
3. *Home care*, a more recently emerging interest dominated by about ten corporate providers.
4. *Laboratory and other services*, another multibillion dollar business growing at a rate of about 15 percent a year. This service, dominated by large corporate providers, packages such health "products" as hospital emergency services, long-term hemo-

dialysis, mobile CAT scanning, cardiopulmonary testing, alcohol and drug abuse programs, and prepaid health maintenance organizations.

Although proprietary hospitals and nursing homes have shared in the lower-profit character of the hospital and nursing home industries in general, it should be noted that proprietary hospitals have made great strides in improving their profitability (Buchanan, 1982).

According to Starr (1982), "the change goes beyond the increased penetration of profit-making firms directly into medical services" (p. 429). Starr has identified five separate dimensions characterizing the change in the health care industry:

1. *Change in type of ownership and control*: the shift from nonprofit and governmental organizations to for-profit companies in health care;
2. *Horizontal integration*: the decline of freestanding institutions and rise of multiinstitutional systems, and the consequent shift in the locus of control from community boards to regional and national health care corporations;
3. *Diversification and corporate restructuring*: the shift from single-unit organizations operating in one market to "polycorporate" and conglomerate enterprises, often organized under holding companies, sometimes with both nonprofit and for-profit subsidiaries involved in a variety of different health care markets;
4. *Vertical integration*: the shift from single-level-of-care organizations, such as acute-care hospitals, to organizations that embrace the various phases and levels of care, such as HMO's;
5. *Industry concentration*: the increasing concentration of ownership and control of health services in regional markets and in the nation as a whole.

Today, about twenty-five multihospital systems own or manage over 50 percent of all community hospitals in the United States (Ricardo-Campbell, 1982, p. 81). The two largest chains are Humana and Hospital Corporation of America. In addition, the for-profit hospitals now comprise about one-third of all hospitals and about one-fifth of acute, general care hospitals (Ricardo-Campbell, 1982, p. 77). However, as one economist has observed, many nonprofit hospitals are managed under contract by profit-making corporations whose primary consideration is financial well-being, not good patient care (Ricardo-Campbell, 1982, p. 82).

Nursing home care constitutes a significant portion of the health dollar spent by and for the aging. The present nursing home industry, with 55 percent of its total revenues from government (Gibson, Waldo, and Levit, 1983), is a product of public policy. It is a multibillion-dollar business in the United States. Capital investment in nursing homes has stimulated the private sector in such industries as construction, banking, business, and drug and medical supplies. It has provided jobs, albeit low paying and nonunion, to over half a million people. In 1980 there were about 23,000 nursing homes serving 1.3 million residents. Most of the residents were old and disabled. The growth of the industry brought total expenditures in 1982 to $27.3 billion, representing 8.5 percent of total health expenditures (Gibson, Waldo, and Levit, 1983).

One in five people living past the age of 65 will spend some time in a nursing home (Vladeck, 1980). If the demand continues at its current rate, there will be a need for 2.5 millon nursing home beds in the United States by 1985, or an increase of 90 percent in the number of beds built between 1976 and 1985. Assuming the cost of nursing home beds continues at its current growth rate, the costs for such growth were projected to be a total of $45 billion of the total estimated $462 billion health expenditures (Freeland and Schendler, 1981).

Home health services constitute a very small share of the health care dollar. Although home health has been a Medicare benefit for some time, this service did not begin to grow until the mid-1970s. Some have predicted that the enactment of the 1980 amendments to Medicare (effective July 1, 1981) would be an incentive to a period of accelerated growth during the 1980s. These amendments eliminated several restrictions: the 100-day visit limitation under Part A, the $60 deductible for home health benefits under Part B, and the 3-day prior hospital stay requirement under Part A. In addition, the amendments have allowed proprietary home health agencies to be Medicare-certified in states without authorizing licensure laws (twenty-six states have such laws) (U.S. Senate, 1982a). Home health has become one of the fastest growing components of federal health expenditures of recent date. By the end of the fiscal year 1980, total expenditures were about $1 billion, with the largest increases occurring in Medicare. In fiscal year 1980, Medicare reimbursement for home health services was $735 million, a fivefold increase since 1974. (U.S. Senate, 1982b). The Inspector General's service delivery assessment of Medicare's home health program observed that there was growing competition among the five major types of providers in home health:

> The two traditional types of providers—visiting nursing associations (VNA's) and public health departments—are challenged by private non-profit, hospital-based, and proprietary providers. The latter three have accounted for nearly all the growth that has occurred in home health agencies. (U.S. Senate, 1982, p. 378)

A major strategy for restructuring the health care industry centers on the health maintenance organization (HMO). HMO's bring a range of health care services from preventative care to acute hospitalization together into a coordinated system with a mandate to maintain its clients' health. Prepayment at a set rate is assumed to ensure that those enrolled will receive adequate medical care in the most cost-efficient form. "With a fixed payment per enrollee, the HMO's net income is inversely related to the number of services provided, and there is a financial incentive to reduce the number of unnecessary procedures" (Luft, 1981, p. 2). Since the HMO assumes at least much of the financial risks of acute care, it is assumed to have an incentive to provide effective preventative care.

Whether or not HMO's do, in fact, emphasize prevention, remains a question. The adequacy of HMO care for the aged is another concern. HMO's do not at present provide long-term nursing home care, nor do they provide the continuum of social services that constitutes an alternative to institutionalization. Moreover, until recently, HMO's have tended not to market to the aged.

Because HMO's appear to be more cost-efficient than conventional health care insurance, they represent competition for traditional health care providers and insurers. It is less clear, however, whether HMO's can provide lower-cost services of adequate quality to the aged and poor recipients of public programs (U.S. General Accounting Office, 1982; Luft, 1981).

HMO's may play an important role in shifting the health industry toward for-profit operations. Although many HMO's were originally set up as nonprofit organizations, they have been taken over increasingly by for-profit firms. In some cases they have been combined into interstate organizations that can compete successfully with traditional providers (Salmon, 1982; Starr, 1982). Starr (1982, p. 439) has concluded that, "without extensive government aid for start-up capital, the consumer-run cooperative organizations are certain to decline, and the surviving HMO's will increasingly become part of large corporate networks." These developments may guarantee that the HMO will be a major instrument in the restructuring of the health care industries along competitive, for-profit lines (see Salmon, 1982; Starr, 1982).

Overview

The rapidly growing health care industry in the United States in the wider view is creating strains on the economic system and in the narrow view is creating a financial burden on governments through their payments for health services. These strains hit simultaneously with increasing fiscal problems of governments at all levels and a recession in the general economy. Possible responses include cutbacks in services or reimbursements, shifting of costs onto consumers, reforms in government reimbursement systems, and alterations in the structure of the health care system itself to accord better with a competitive, for-profit model.

Whether or not these trends continue, and whether or not the responses adequately address the problems, the question arises as to how these problems will affect the aged. The competition model as a prescription for the nation's health care woes is aimed at restricting access to health care, and it is doubtful that it will ensure quality of care. The shifting of greater costs onto consumers will more likely limit access to needed services for those with less ability to pay than make the services fit "real" needs. The use of the voucher or other "consumer choice" plans for government subsidy of services for the needy is likely only to ensure that the poor will receive bare-bones health plans, while those with the ability to pay for more comprehensive plans will enjoy better coverage (Salmon, 1982). Moreover, the shift from public investment to financially autonomous models means that the question will increasingly be one of the profitability, rather than the availability, of services offered.

Although the present system involves duplication of services, sometimes of doubtful value to those receiving them, the competitive health care model may feature the withholding of needed services and the rationing of the services offered. Salmon has suggested that those with "less valuable 'human capital' and the nonworking population . . . may find their care further restricted, quality neglected and costlier services denied" (1982, p. 29). Insofar as the elderly are nonworking and are financially dependent, these effects are likely to fall heavily on them. The rapid increases in copayments and deductibles in the Medicare system have already set the pace. Likewise, those elders in nursing homes are overwhelmingly in for-profit homes. They already face rationing of needed levels of care, particularly skilled care, as Medicaid and other government reimbursement competes less successfully with private reimbursement. Further and accelerated trends in the direction of the competitive health care model do not bode well for the aged.

Chapter

5

The Social Creation
of Dependency

In mid-1983, the mayor of the town of Santa Clara, in the heart of California's prosperous Silicon Valley, publicly berated elderly people who did not have the "foresight to save some money" and who came "begging" to local government for handouts. This kind of outburst, rarely heard in a public setting, reflects an ideological perspective that has produced contemporary health, social, and economic programs for the aged. Preceding chapters have described the value conflicts and political environment that have shaped the way old age health care is delivered in the context of U.S. economic requirements. In this chapter, we turn to look at the effects of lifelong social and economic conditions on the health status of older persons. In describing the actual health and economic situation of elders, we are pointing to what Alan Walker (1981, p. 49) calls "the social creation of poverty and dependency in old age." Old people as a group are not impoverished because of lack of foresight, but because the economy is organized around differential rewards for productive labor, from which they are in large part excluded. The labeling of legitimate political demands and lobbying efforts by older people as begging is a failure to recognize the ways in which health policy, programs, and services have placed elders in a position of collective dependency.

Dependency can be a matter of social definition, of society's defining and treating an individual as dependent, and a matter of self-definition, of seeing oneself as helpless, powerless, or needy (Munnichs and van den Heuvel, 1976). Dependency is commonly treated in the literature as a function of individual lifetime choices about education, work skills, occupation, savings, and economic resources (Clark and Spengler, 1980). This says nothing, however, about the social context of dependency. Dependency "always has reference to a social relationship in which it occurs" (Munnichs and van den Heuvel, 1976, p. 165). Although negative connotations of dependency are deeply rooted in the national psyche, the phenomenon of dependency is not necessarily undesirable. Mutual dependence is necessary to form and maintain human relationships. Munnichs and van den Heuvel (1976), for example, find interdependency more descriptive of "the concrete situation in which many people find themselves than the polar extremes of independence or dependence" (p. 4).

There is no single reason why old age dependency is perceived as a problem for society. The effects of aging that create dependency may be divided into biological and social factors. The biological effects of aging cause wear and tear on the body's mental and physical state (primary aging) and may threaten independent functioning. Although the biochemistry of cell and hormonal changes related to aging has been the subject of intensive study, we have no sure explanations for the mechanisms of these processes. The fact that these changes happen within individuals at different rates renders chronological age an inadequate measure of physiological age. Consequently, generalizations made about the physical and mental health of age groups are of uncertain validity. The social effects of aging (secondary aging), which also affect health status, must be considered in assessing dependency status (Hickey, 1980). Often grouped under the rubric of the social environment, social factors include personal lifestyle, family support, education, habits, and nutrition. These factors have the potential to be controlled by the individual. Other social factors include elements of the physical environment—chemical exposure, air and water impurity, occupational hazards, consumer product safety, risks of nuclear accidents, and so on.

Health and social policy interventions have largely focused on those factors that can be changed by the exercise of individual choice. In contrast, the politicoeconomic context of aging and health, while potentially subject to intervention, is not easily affected by individual action. Walker's (1980) analysis of the social creation of dependency in old age underscores the point that many complex social and political forces are called into play. Myles concurs, in the sense that:

"Old people" as we now know them are an *effect*, not a cause of the welfare state. Withdrawal from the labor force in advance of physiological old age—the institutionalization of retirement and the creation of a new social category of superannuated elders, especially within the working class—occurred after and was made possible by the invention of old age pensions and other welfare state programs. (1981, p. 7)

Economic and Social Well-Being

It is particularly useful in disentangling this complex web of social forces to distinguish three groups of the aged: first, those aged 55–64; second, those aged 65–74; and third, those aged 75 and over (Storey, 1983). Social forces influencing dependency vary with the distinct social relations found within these different age groups.

The 55–64 Group. For the first group, aged 55 to 64, economic growth and participation in the labor market is critical in determining social and economic well-being. The dynamics of the labor market, including monetary and fiscal policy, business cycle downturns, and age and sex discrimination practices, constitute the single most important structural cause of dependency for those in the group aged 55 to 64. For both men and women, exigencies in the labor market during times of recession and stagflation can lead to forced early retirement. Unless one has substantial private investments and large savings (which few older people have) to offset the reduction in Social Security benefits for early retirees and the erosion of retirement savings by inflation, the loss of earnings income can greatly diminish one's financial resources and create sudden dependency on public programs. In Western industrialized countries, dependency may be created at an even earlier age than formal retirement mandates (Guillemard, 1983). For workers aged 55 years and over, withdrawal from the labor market may be caused by adverse economic changes such as urbanization, increased technology, labor competition from younger persons, industry opportunities, and age discrimination. The withdrawal from the labor market is referred to as the discouraged-worker effect and is most prevalent among older workers (Bowen and Finegan, 1969; Cain and Watts, 1973; Rosenblum, 1975). Walker (1980) has encapsulated these phenomena, stating that superannuation functions to carry the social costs of economic and industrial change.

Restricted access to the labor market for older workers, due to age discrimination, recession layoffs, or restricted job supply, affects their disposable income and health status. There is a large body of research linking swings in the business cycle, unemployment, and physical and mental illness (Brenner, 1976; Eyer, 1976a; 1976b; Luft, 1978). In studying the linkage between health problems and economic fluctuations, Brenner (1973) found, over a 127-year period, significant correlations between the economy and almost all categories of mental hospital admissions. Economic downturns have also been shown to be related to mortality caused by cirrhosis of the liver, cardiovascular disease, and renal disease (Brenner, 1975a; 1975b).

The labor market experience has particular effects on economic status and dependency for women. Over the past thirty years, there has been an enormous increase in labor force participation by older women (Kreps and Clark, 1975; Olson, Caton, and Duffy, 1981). Women comprise about 40 percent of the labor force aged 45 and over, compared with 25 percent in 1950 (M.I.T., 1973). The dramatic alteration in the composition of the older labor force in the United States can be attributed to many factors: women's changing role in society, economics, the growth of the service sector including the health care industry, increased education, and political pressures for equal opportunities in employment (Ross and Birdsall, 1980; Urquhart, 1981). The experience of women in the labor force, however, is often characterized by low-wage occupations, uneven employment, and differential pay for work comparable to that done by men. Many of the issues of inequity in Social Security benefits for older women are linked to these employment problems.

One of the traditional roles for women that has not changed is that of primary caregiver. Often such phrases as "the family" or "the informal support system" are euphemisms for women as the primary caregivers responding to the long-term care needs of family members (Brody, 1981). Married or unmarried women are often "called to duty" to take care of their chronically ill spouses, parents, or parents-in-law. This may require reentry into the labor market at a later age in order to make up for the loss of the spouse's income, or an early withdrawal from the labor market in order to provide care at home. If a spouse must enter a nursing home, income and resources (including any nest egg for old age) are treated as communal. Both the husband and wife are required to "spend down" their assets and income in order to be eligible for long-term public support. The overall effect of stress, social isolation, and restricted financial and emotional resources also can place the caregiver, frequently an older woman, at risk of illness. Thus, a woman's role as caregiver in a family unit may be transformed into that of patient or beneficiary dependent on the state.

The 65–74 Group. For the second group, aged 65 to 74, mandatory retirement is the most critical social institution affecting dependency status, primarily because it reduces an individual's income by approximately one-half (Brotman, 1982). Historically, the introduction of mandatory retirement in the United States around the turn of the century has posed the gravest threat to financial security in old age. The increasing demand for mandatory retirement was fueled by the exigencies of an economy with episodic unemployment and the need for a means of transferring skills generationally in industries with surplus labor (Graebner, 1980). The concept and policy of superannuating older workers helped to identify the elderly with dependency. Old age came to be associated with physical decline and lowered productivity, with the consequent idea that labor market opportunities should be restricted to a more youthful and vigorous population.

Although the effects of a lifelong social class membership persist into older age and are reflected in the broad range of economic resources of elderly individuals, income is compressed toward the lower end of the scale among those whose major financial resources came from wages or salary. The poverty rate of older persons has risen dramatically from 14 percent in 1978 to 15.7 percent (or 3.9 million people) in 1980. More significantly, there is a larger percentage of persons over 65 who are stacked just above the official poverty threshold. If the near poor (those with incomes between 125 and 150 percent of the current poverty criteria) are considered, the poverty rate increases to 35 percent (Lehrman, 1980). Women, blacks, and other minorities are the most disadvantaged, with 38 percent of aged blacks and 30.8 percent of aged Hispanics living at extreme poverty levels (Brotman, 1982). Moreover, half of all the aged poor are single women (women who have never married or widows) who live alone (Orshansky in U.S. House, 1978). While it is estimated that Social Security preserves two-thirds of the older population from acute poverty, it is still insufficient to keep millions of retired persons from near poverty (U.S. General Accounting Office, 1981). The median income of people 65 and older in the United States in 1980 was $4,226, which is approximately half of the median income of younger adults (Storey, 1983).

Given these low income levels, the failure to adjust for increases in the cost of living directly affects the amount of disposable income for the majority of older persons. For example, between 1974 and 1980, real income for the aged declined 7 to 8 percent for older married couples and 3 to 4 percent for older unmarried individuals (U.S. Senate, Special Committee on Aging, 1982a).

The 75+ Group. The oldest group, aged 75 years and over, is most vulnerable to poverty because of its dependency on public resources and programs to offset social factors such as diminished finances, loss of spouse or family supports, urban relocation, and increased incidence of health problems. Table 5-1 shows the decrease in income from labor market earnings by age. The percentage of aged who are 75 years and older, now comprising 38 percent of the elderly population, is expected to grow to 45 percent by the year 2000 (Duffy et al., 1980; Townsend, 1979; U.S. General Accounting Office, 1981). By the year 2000 it is estimated that two-thirds of those over 75 will be women (U.S. National Institute on Aging, 1979). The

Table 5-1
Percent of Aged Units (Individuals and Couples) with Earnings from
Employment in 1980

Age	Percent
55–61	81
62–64	62
65–67	45
68–72	27
73–79	16
80–older	5

Source: Grad, S. *Income of the Population 55 and Over, 1980.* Washington, D.C.: U.S. Government
Printing Office, 1983.

factors in public programs that contribute to dependency are
discussed in the final section of this chapter.

Population Growth
and the Dependency Ratio

Parallel to the increasing financial dependency of older people has
been an increase in the proportion of aged people in the population.
More than 25 million people are 65 and over according to the 1980
U.S. census. This represents 11.3 percent of the total population, up
from less than 3 percent a century ago when the first compulsory
retirement policies were introduced. Although the elderly comprise
only 11.3 percent of the population, nearly one-third of health
expenditures go for their care. In 1980, the per capita health
expenditure for older people was over $2,500, compared to $710 for
members of the younger population (Rice, 1983).

Alarm over disproportionate population growth of the aged and
the social costs of their care has focused attention on the ratio of
persons of working age (18 to 64) to those of nonworking age (young
people under 18 and old people over 64). This ratio, called the
"dependency ratio," reflects the fact that goods and services allocated
to those who are still in school or retired must be produced and
supported by the working population. How much is available is
conditioned by the size of the working population, its average
productivity, the wage and price structure, and the willingness of its
working members to assume taxes to finance the costs of supporting
retired persons (Clark and Spengler, 1980).

Concern has been expressed over the increasing ratio of elders to those who are 18 to 64. This ratio is expected to increase from approximately 19 per 100 in 1980 to nearly 32 per 100 in 2030, when the last of the baby boomers reach 65 (Brotman, 1982). However, the total dependency ratio (the number of youth and elders combined compared to the working population) will actually be *reduced*, when comparing the ratio for 1970 and those projected for the years 2000 and 2050. In other words, barring unforeseen events, there will be *fewer* dependents per worker in the next century than there were between 1950 and 1970.

Health and Social Class

The relationship between class and health involves issues related to the etiology of disease and probability of death, to the access to treatment and the quality of care received, as well as to the differential occupational health risks that have direct and long-lasting influence on health status. The social and economic situations of elders, both past and current, are major determinants of their ability to maintain physical well-being and independence. On the whole, elders persist in the ability to have productive lives long after they are socially discredited from being able to do so.

Mortality

Studies of the effects of social class membership on health have shown consistently that lower class status predicts shorter life expectancy and higher death rates from all diseases (Antonovsky, 1967; Kitagawa and Hauser, 1973). These findings have been substantiated repeatedly despite inconsistencies in methodologies, populations studied, historical periods, and measures of social class. Traditionally, income, level of education, occupation, or some combination of the three have been used as indicators of social class. Kitagawa and Hauser (1973) found all three indicators of class, considered separately or together, to vary with mortality rates in adults aged 25 to 64. They found that males with the lowest family incomes had a 49 percent higher mortality rate than the general white male population, while those with the highest incomes had a 16 percent lower death rate. This relationship held true for white women as well, though the degree of difference was not as striking.

Mortality rates vary greatly among races in the United States, although rates for nonwhites have declined at a faster pace (Davis and

Table 5-2
Life Expectancy at Birth and at Age 65 by Race and Sex: United States, 1979

	At birth			At age 65		
	White	All others	Total	White	All others	Total
Male	70.6	65.5	69.9	14.2	14.4	14.2
Female	78.2	74.2	77.6	18.7	18.4	18.6
Both sexes	74.4	69.8	73.7	16.6	16.5	16.6

Source: U.S. Department of Health and Human Services, Public Health Service. *Health: United States.* Washington, D.C.: U.S. Government Printing Office, 1982, p. 53.

Schoen, 1978). Block (1979) has cited an average life expectancy of only 44 years for American Indians. Life expectancy for people of Japanese or Chinese heritage, however, is higher than for the general population (Rudov and Santangelo, 1979). Life expectancies at birth and at age 65 for whites and all others by sex are shown in Table 5-2. There is a difference of about four to five years of longevity at birth between whites and nonwhites, but life expectancy at age 65 is approximately equivalent.

Manton (1982) has argued that, within higher-risk cohorts (for example, low-income, working class, or black), life expectancy at age 65 corresponds more closely to that of the general population because higher-risk members of the cohort are more likely to die prior to reaching old age. Comparison of age-specific mortality rates from heart disease, by sex for instance, show that the greatest excess mortality occurs prior to old age for blacks (see Table 5-3). Both black males and females have greatly elevated risks of dying from coronary heart disease, compared to same-sex whites of the same age cohort, prior to age 65. For black males, comparative risk drops dramatically in old age. While risk continues to be greater for black women than white women through age 84, differences between the two groups diminish. Longitudinal data are needed to analyze the crossover of mortality risks among subgroups of the population, although cross-sectional data lend credence to Manton's explanation that early deaths in high-risk populations account for the diminution of racial differences in mortality risk in old age.

Morbidity

Morbidity is highly related to mortality, although the nature of their relationship in old age is debated. Fries (1980) has postulated a biological limit for the human life-span, arguing that observed mortality reductions and life expectancy increases will not continue. Control over chronic disease through personal responsibility for disease prevention will diminish premature death, so that people will live healthfully throughout most of their allotted 85 years, dying of senescence rather than disease. Disease will be compressed toward the very end of life. Kramer (1980) and Gruenberg (1977) have disagreed with Fries, predicting that longer life-spans will result from the control of the deadly outcomes of chronic disease. However, people will live with chronic disease for more extended periods, and prevalence of morbidity in the population (the number of sick people at any given time) will be higher. This will place even greater demands on the health system.

Table 5-3
Mortality Ratios for Heart Disease by Race, Sex and Age: United States, 1979

	All ages (age adjusted)	45–54	55–64	65–74	75–84	85–over
Total	100	100	100	100	100	100
White male	138	151	148	143	128	119
White female	66	39	50	65	83	99
Black male	157	225	191	143	129	66
Black female	99	112	106	94	103	55

Note: Ratios reflect the proportion of the death rate in the subgroup population to the death rate of the population as a whole within each age group.
Source: Adapted from U.S. Department of Health and Human Services, Public Health Service. *Health: United States.* Washington, D.C.: U.S. Government Printing Office, December, 1982, pp. 61–62.

Based on population statistics, Manton (1982) has challenged both points of view. He argued that recent accretions in the life-span among the very old belie assertions of a ceiling on potential life-span. Between 1960 and 1978, life expectancy for white females at age 85 increased two years, and for nonwhite females, four and one-half years. Census figures for 1982 indicate the presence of over 32,000 centenarians in the United States. Furthermore, Health Interview Survey data for older people show no evidence of increased prevalence of morbidity or disability over the last two decades. Manton has suggested that the disease-free life-span is increasing and that individual age-related disability occurs more rapidly and closer to death than cohort or cross-sectional data appear to suggest.

> The weight of this evidence indicates that not only is the rate of aging highly variable among individuals, but that our stereotype of elderly persons seriously underestimates their ability to maintain functional capacity at older ages. (Manton, 1982, p. 205)

Manton's analysis is cause for optimism about the projected general health condition of individual older people, but also cause for alarm over continuing increases in the health care costs because of the demographics of aging. Chronic conditions are widespread among the elderly. Of the noninstitutionalized older population, 20 percent have heart conditions, 44 percent have arthritis, 20 percent have hypertension, and 29 percent have a hearing impairment (Rice and Feldman, 1983). These conditions and their effects, however, are not randomly distributed among elders.

In 1979, almost half (46 percent) of noninstitutionalized people 65 and over reported chronic activity limitation. Nearly 17 percent stated that they were unable to work or keep house, and another 22 percent claimed limitation in the amount or kind of work they could do. Table 5-4 shows these limitations of activity due to chronic conditions by income, race, and education for those 65 and over. Data from Table 5-4 complement the social class–health status findings related to mortality, which were presented earlier. Activity limitation accompanying chronic condition is greater for those in lower-income and lower-education groups, and for those who are nonwhite.

Self-Care Limitations

The most extreme form of activity limitation is the inability to perform activities of daily living (ADL), such as bathing and dressing oneself, eating, and going to the toilet. Inability to care for oneself physically on a day-to-day basis is the most salient form of depen-

Table 5-4
Percent of Population Aged 65 and Over with Limitations of
Activity Due to Chronic Conditions by Family Income, Race, and
Education: United States, 1974

	Percent with limitation
Total family income	
less than $3,000	54.9
$3,000–$4,999	49.1
$5,000–$6,999	43.1
$7,000–$9,999	40.3
$10,000–$14,999	41.4
$15,000 or more	38.4
Race and family income	
white	44.8
less than $5,000	50.8
$5,000 or more	40.8
all other	56.2
less than $5,000	59.9
$5,000 or more	45.5
Educational attainment	
less than 5 years	61.2
5–8 years	49.0
9–11 years	43.7
12 years	37.4
13–15 years	38.4
16 years or more	34.2

Source: U.S. Dept. of Health, Education, and Welfare, Nat'l. Center for Health Statistics Series 10, Number 111, 1977, pp. 5–6.

Table 5-5
Percent of Persons with Activity Limitation, and Persons
Dependent in Various Activities of Daily Living (ADL) by Age:
United States Noninstitutional, 1977

Age	45–64	65–74	74–84	85 and over
With activity limitation	23.0	38.6	48.4	63.2
Dependent in at least one ADL	0.7	2.2	5.8	15.0
Dependent in all four ADL's	0.08	0.4	0.6	3.7

Source: Health Care Financing Administration, 1981. Published by American Health Care Financing Administration.

dency. Table 5-5 breaks down by age the noninstitutionalized adult population experiencing chronic activity limitation or dependency in activities of daily living. These data indicate that the vast majority of elders are able to function independently with respect to fulfilling personal daily needs.

Utilization of Health Care

Utilization of health care is another phenomenon affecting health that is highly associated with social class. Kleinman, Gold, and Makuc (1981) analyzed National Health Interview Survey (NHIS) data for 1976 to 1978 and found that impoverished people have higher absolute health service utilization rates. However, instituting controls for health status (self-perception of comparative health condition) and age alters the relationship between income and utilization. Table 5-6 shows that of those reporting poor or fair health, impoverished elders of both races make 25 percent fewer visits to physicians than do those in the highest income group and that blacks make 15 percent fewer visits than do whites. These relationships do not hold for those reporting good or excellent health (that is, healthy blacks and whites have similar health care utilization patterns). Aday and Andersen (1981), also using NHIS data, found fewer visits to physicians for the poor elderly than for the nonpoor elderly when health status was controlled. In 1979, the ratio of visits to physicians per 100 disability days for poor to nonpoor was .61 (that is, poor elderly saw a physician less than two-thirds as often as nonpoor elderly did). When ratios were adjusted for chronic illness, the ratio of visits to physicians for poor to nonpoor was .90.

While most elderly are eligible for Medicare, research has shown that more Medicare benefits are provided to the upper and middle

Table 5-6
Estimated Number of Physician Visits per Person per Year for Those Aged 65 or Older Reporting Poor or Fair Health by Race and Income, 1976–1978

Income	White	Black
Below poverty level	8.90	7.58
100–150% of poverty level	9.61	8.18
150–200% of poverty level	10.66	9.08
Above 200% of poverty level	11.90	10.14

Source: Adapted from Kleinman, Gold, and Makuc (1981), p. 1016.

classes and to whites than are provided to lower classes and to blacks (Davis, 1975). Inequities in Medicare benefits are associated with income, race, and region. In the southern region of the United States, where 56 percent of the nation's aged nonwhites reside, the disparities between white and nonwhite Medicare beneficiaries persist (Ruther and Dobson, 1981). Further, aged of the upper and middle classes can afford to supplement these benefits with private health insurance, and they are better able to meet the increasing cost of copayments and deductibles under Medicare than are the aged of the lower classes.

In short, wealth and its distribution in the nation enormously affect the capacity to maintain health. Wealth provides greater opportunities for rest, sound nutrition, education, emotional security, lack of stress, and status as well as greater capacity to have illness treated (Butler and Lewis, 1982). Certainly the amount of disposable income available to older persons influences important individual choices concerning independence and well-being. For these reasons, it can be argued strongly that improving the income of older persons may be the most beneficial health policy strategy (Ball, 1981; McKinlay and McKinlay, 1977).

Theories on the Relationship of Class and Health

The universal association of mortality and morbidity rates with low income or minority racial group identity raises important but unanswered questions about the underlying phenomena that can explain these trends. Disease-specific hypotheses do not address why this relationship exists for nearly every disease. Differential exposure to a noxious physical environment also does not account for the universal nature of the inverse relationship between class and health status (Syme and Berkman, 1976). Furthermore, there is some controversy about the effect of improved medical care quality and access on adult health status in the United States (McKinlay and McKinlay, 1977; Hadley, 1982).

Historically, medicine has moved from single-cause explanations of disease, such as the germ theory, to multiple-cause explanations, such as the effects of diet, smoking, and exercise on heart disease. Najman (1980) has described elements of a more encompassing explanation—the concept of "general susceptibility," a term coined by Syme and Berkman. One appealing theory that seems to have broad generalizable applicability is posed by Cassel (1974), who views susceptibility to disease as a function of both exposure to stressors in the environment and possession of protective buffers against the stressors. Acknowledging individual variation in reaction to given stress situations, Cassel suggested examining similarities in social circumstances within a given culture or subculture to identify common responses to stress. Further, he cited animal and human studies to indicate that "the property common to protective processes is the strength of the social supports provided by the primary groups of most importance to the individual" (p. 58).

Health and Social Policy and Dependency

The role of social and family support in assisting older people to maintain an independent status in life has been an important subject of social epidemiology (McGaugh and Kiesler, 1981). Kane and Kane (1982) also have pointed to the continued exercise of control and choice in one's life as critical factors in maintaining an independent and healthy state of well-being. To this end, incentives in public programs that favor particular types of health policy and services for the elderly are an important dimension in understanding how dependency may be socially established.

There are three environments or settings in which health and social services are rendered: closed (institutional), open (community), and unorganized (informal/home) (Little, 1982). The boundaries between the three sectors are not static, but rather are subject to shifting definitions and funding patterns. Table 5-7 shows the organization of care and funding for each sector. The critical variable in this conceptualization of health and social services is the degree of power and status conferred on the elderly within the structure of each setting (Little, 1982).

Health and social welfare programs can have an intended or unintended impact on the unorganized informal sector. The method and means of financing and the scope of services covered follow a complex pattern and, more importantly, interact in very critical ways. Income maintenance programs such as Social Security can affect the amount of services in a closed or open setting. The unorganized or informal sector currently provides the major portion of care (Brody, 1981; Little, 1982; Filner and Williams, 1981). Programs and services in the open setting are aimed at maintaining an independent life in the community. We find, however, that throughout the world, regardless of ideology and political system, open care is less developed and less funded than is care in the closed sector (Little, 1982). The closed or institutional setting, which is the most restrictive, consumes the lion's share of public funds for the elderly in the United States. For example, while 86 percent of the Medicaid dollar for the elderly in 1981 went to hospitals and nursing homes, 1.2 percent was spent on home or community health services. Similarly, although Medicare is

Table 5-7
The Organization of Care

Type of setting	Major type of service	Source of payment
Closed institutional	Acute care hospital, psychiatric hospital, nursing homes (SNF/ICF)	Medicare and Medicaid
Open community	Health services: home health, adult day, community mental health	Medicare and/or Medicaid
	Social services: senior centers, nutrition sites, transportation, homemaker	Social services block grant, Older Americans Act
	Board and care homes: domiciliary, residential group, and other private homes or hotels	Supplementary Security Income, private
Informal/ unorganized home	Variable: may require no care or a lot; degrees of care provided largely by family, spouse, children, friends or individual may be self-sufficient	Social Security, private pensions, tax policies, income from employment, assets and other private sources, Supplementary Security Income

Source: Table adapted from Little, V. *Open Care for the Aging*. New York: Springer, 1982.

the primary source of funding for home health services, less than 2 percent of the total Medicare budget in 1982 was expended on home health services (Harrington, 1983). Thus the discrepancy between those services that appear on paper and those that are, in actuality, available and accessible to those seeking care at a particular time is still a very real problem.

Health care policy has been criticized for its high cost, its fragmentation, its bias toward acute rather than chronic illness, and its emphasis on institutional solutions (in that it finances hospital and nursing home care) (Kane and Kane, 1981; 1982; Butler and Lewis, 1982). Health and social policy define which of the needs of the sick and aged will be addressed. The dominant response to meeting those needs has been a service policy of institutionalization, primarily in nursing homes, as reflected by an increase of 267 percent in the proportion of elderly people residing in institutions and group quarters of one type or another between 1910 and 1970 (Estes and Harrington, 1981). The combination of poverty, loss of social status and social supports, and chronic illness has forced growing numbers of aged into institutional confinement. Although income, housing, and social policies are of great importance to the elderly, it has been the Medicare financing of hospital and physician services and Medicaid financing of nursing home care that have dominated public policy for the aged.

Long-term care may ideally be conceptualized as a mix of personal, health, housing, and social services and income support. However, the availability of financing for institutional care has resulted in nursing home care's being the de facto long-term care policy in the United States. Between 1975 and 1980, spending for nursing home care almost doubled. In 1980, nursing home care totaled $20.7 billion, or 8.4 percent of the total national health care expenditures (Gibson and Waldo, 1981). By the year 1990, it is estimated that the United States will spend in excess of $75 billion on all aspects of nursing home care (Butler and Lewis, 1982).

The human needs of the aged who are marginally poor or financially destitute and suffering from ill health are often dealt with by the government in the context of the prevailing political environment. Both Durkheim and Marx identified inequities in the "distribution of resources and power as the major mechanism by which individuals' options are differentially limited and controlled" (Williamson, 1982, p. 218). Thus, institutionalization serves social ends. It substitutes medically defined services at a profit for adequate housing and income policies and controls the behavior of the poor and sick. As Townsend (1981) has pointed out, part of the social control function of institutions is "to regulate deviation from the central social values of self-help, domestic independence, personal thrift, willingness to work, productive effort and family care" (pp. 21–22). Eligibility for public assistance for long-term care in nursing homes requires liquidating all but a very small portion of assets, virtually guaranteeing permanent poverty status for beneficiaries. What we observe are trade-offs between public order and security, on the one hand, and personal autonomy on the other.

Many individuals have been placed in institutions primarily because they lack the social and economic support necessary for independent living (Butler and Newacheck, 1981; U.S. General Accounting Office, 1979). A brief review of the utilization trends of different types of institutional care reveals the mutable and arbitrary definitions of need, diagnosis, and placement. Haber (1983) has described the treatment of the aged during the nineteenth century, indicating that most physicians "seemed convinced of the chronicity of mental disease in the aged," with little or no objective medical criteria (p. 90). Those who became dependent because of age and illness were placed in mental asylums (Haber, 1983). This practice continued well into the twentieth century and even up until the early 1960s; the elderly poor and sick were shunted into state mental institutions that functioned as custodial warehouses (not unlike the English Poor Law almshouses).

Examining the relationship of socioeconomic status to state mental hospital referrals of the elderly in 1967–1968, Markson and Hand (1970) found that the disproportionate number of lower-income aged who were referred to state hospitals could not be attributed to a higher rate of mental illness in the group. For reasons associated with the combined effect of social class and loss of social roles, poor old people were especially liable to placement in state mental hospitals when sick, whether or not they were mentally ill. Another study comparing institutionalization for blacks and whites in twenty-six states (Kart and Beckham, 1976) found substantial differences. Blacks were overrepresented in state mental hospitals, and whites were overrepresented in proprietary nursing homes. Although data were inconclusive in correlating utilization with actual mental health status, socioeconomic factors and racial discrimination accounted for some of these variations between blacks and whites.

The wholesale shift in care of the elderly poor from mental facilities to hospitals and nursing homes was the result of Medicare and Medicaid, which began to provide federal support for hospitals and nursing homes in 1965. In most cases, before Medicare and Medicaid the state governments had carried the full cost of placement in mental institutions. When Medicaid was enacted, states began to shift patients out of mental hospitals and into nursing homes because partial federal funding was provided for the latter (Holahan, 1975). States also shifted some of the fiscal burden of the aged and mentally ill to the federal government by using the Supplemental Security Income (SSI) program. SSI made it possible for older persons to pay for board and care, supporting the growth of another private sector profit-making industry. The deinstitutionalization of state and county mental hospitals was severely criticized because, in many cases, alternative programs were not provided to those patients "dumped" from public institutions (Clarke, 1979). Many aged were forced to move to substandard, totally unregulated boarding homes or old hotels, while others lived on the streets (U.S. Senate, 1974–1976).

Whether these wholesale shifts of patients from mental institutions to nursing and boarding homes were a move for the better is a matter of contention. The point is that definitions of need, diagnosis, and placement have been determined by social policy and its financing (Vladeck, 1980; Dunlop, 1979). Studies comparing patients in nursing homes to those in the community report little difference in characteristics between the two groups for one-third of those in nursing homes. State and federal policy has been skewed toward the financing of institutional facilities and acute medical care in hospitals. There has been little incentive to meet the health and social needs of those aged with chronic or debilitating illnesses in any way other than nursing homes. Further, profit incentives under present reimbursement systems encourage the selection of patients who need relatively less nursing and personal care, and the rejection of those who require heavy nursing care because such care is more costly. Therefore, the rates of inappropriate placement are high—ranging from 5 to 75 percent, depending on the criteria used (U.S. Senate, 1974–1976; U.S. General Accounting Office, 1979; Liu and Mossey, 1980).

A persistent issue in the public and private debate on long-term care and the elderly concerns the consequences of medical care in the context of quality of care (Vladeck, 1980; 1981a; Newcomer and Harrington, 1983; Koff, 1982). Medical iatrogenesis, the creation of illness as a product of medical treatment, is largely a symptom of a system that allocates profits through institutional solutions fostering dependency, passivity, and acquiescence. Countries with fewer resources than the United States have done more to maintain the elderly in a state of maximum independence (Kane and Kane, 1982).

The use and misuse of drugs by the elderly exemplifies the more general problem of adverse effects of medical treatment. Lee and Lipton (1982) have observed:

> The consumption of prescription and over-the-counter drugs by the elderly is an almost universal phenomenon. Not only is drug use influenced by the prevalence of illness and disability among the elderly, but it is influenced by a host of nonillness factors, as well: mass media advertising, self care practices learned within the family or social group, family size, percentage of females in the family, sex, family income, age, physician-patient relationship, access to medical care, and insurance coverage for prescription drugs. (p. 15)

Numerous studies have shown that among the elderly, especially those in nursing homes, there is an extraordinary consumption of drugs (Prentice, 1979; Stephens, Haney, and Underwood, 1982; Eve and Friedsam, 1982). Over 95 percent of the elderly in nursing homes receive drugs, with estimates in one study being an average of six drugs per resident per day. Many psychoactive drugs are widely used in nursing homes for patient management problems rather than for any therapeutic value (Lee and Lipton, 1982).

The nation's noninstitutionalized elderly also utilize prescription drugs at a higher rate than do those under 65 (Lee and Lipton, 1982; Fisher, 1980). Of those 120 million Americans who received at least one prescription outside the hospital in 1977, the average number of prescriptions was 7.5; for the elderly it was 14.2 (Kasper,

1982). Cooper (1981) has estimated that over 80 percent of elderly ambulatory patients take prescription drugs, many of which are psychoactive.

Overview

The long-term care system is characterized by (1) a largely for-profit incentive with an orientation toward institutional medical care, (2) welfare rather than entitlement notions, (3) fee-for-service and cost-related reimbursement policies that foster price inflation, (4) a closed system that restricts the elements of choice once a patient has entered it, and (5) low-prestige careers for those who work in the field (Kane and Kane, 1982). Aged people who are disabled or chronically ill are channeled into an alienating environment in which those unskilled and poorly paid workers who are most marginal to society are in the position of delegated control and management of other marginal members of society, namely their elderly patients. This is particularly noteworthy in nursing homes, whose workers are held in low esteem in the United States. This has been attributed at least partially to our value system, which ascribes the "dirty work" of caring for the old, sick, and poor to other members of society with a devalued status—minorities, recent immigrants, and women (Sclar, 1980; Vladeck, 1980; Kane and Kane, 1982).

Undoubtedly, there have been many positive professional and community efforts directed at a more humane and comprehensive long-term care policy of services and programs. Koff (1982) envisions a long-term care system in which institutionally based and community-based services are integrated and appropriately utilized. However, as we discussed in the preceding chapter, the development of such a continuum of health care for the elderly has been subordinated by the vested interests of the medical-industrial complex. In addition, the economic uncertainty and the political climate of fiscal austerity in the 1980s have added to the pressure on governments to curb health care spending. Unfortunately, expedient cost-cutting measures often supercede the issue of real reform in long-term care health policy (Estes and Newcomer, 1983).

It is indeed difficult to encapsulate the issue of dependency and the health of the elderly in an optimistic summary framework. According to Davis (1981):

> Despite the well-known seriousness of the dependency needs of the elderly and the clear indication that this problem will magnify alarmingly in future years, no major long-term care proposal for the elderly has even

been advanced by any President, seriously debated by the Congress, or received highest priority for public policy action at the federal, state, or local level. (p. 1)

There is no clear consensus as to whether the private or the public sector or as to which level of government should assume the responsibility for long-term care. Even given the many articles, books, and research studies on the topic, long-term care is an issue largely ignored and left to the will of politicians, business entrepreneurs, and voluntary organizations. Yet, as Davis has concluded:

The issue cannot be forgotten. One in five persons reaching the age of 65 will spend some time in a nursing home. It touches families of all incomes, races, and geographical locations. Those elderly who cannot care for themselves have lived lives not unlike our own. They are, indeed, our future selves. (1981, p. 1)

Chapter

6

An Era of Crisis: The Class Basis of Sacrifice

The 1980s are best described as an era of crisis. A crisis mentality pervades the everyday lives of millions of Americans as we receive the wisdom and words of our legislators, our president, our governors, our mayors, business and labor leaders, and fellow citizens through the mass media. Crises in the news include a fiscal crisis, a health care crisis, a deficit crisis, a demographic crisis (in the aging of the population), an education crisis, a productivity crisis, and on and on. Most noteworthy, yet virtually unacknowledged by the purveyors of these various crises, is that each of the crises making their way into the public consciousness is socially "produced," or constructed by what politicians, economists, experts, and the media say about or impute to the issues they address. This is not to deny that real conditions exist that might appropriately be said to constitute crises, however, these conditions are but the stuff of which publicly acknowledged crises may be constructed, given the views and interests of those in positions of power.

National Crises and Aging

Social, economic, and political stakes are invested in the definitions and perceptions of social problems and whether or not the problems are considered to be crises (Edelman, 1977; Estes, 1979). The role that organized interests play in defining a crisis is not always evident, as Edelman has observed:

The long term developments that make it possible for strategically located groups to precipitate a crisis, unintentionally or deliberately, are always complex and ambiguous. People who benefit from a crisis are usually able to explain it to themselves and to the mass public in terms that mask or minimize their own contributions and incentives, while highlighting outside threats and unexpected occurrences. The divergence between the symbolic import of crises and their material impact is basic to their popular acceptance. (1977, p. 46)

Past crises, and the remembrance of them, provide an important impetus for future action; they often permit broad discretion by government. Actions by government that would ordinarily be strongly resisted are often readily accepted by the public in response to a crisis. The labeling of a problem as a crisis does more than denote an undesirable state of affairs; it has many political uses (Edelman, 1964; 1971; 1977; Alford, 1976). Crisis labels marshall both action and sacrifice. They also imply that the event or condition is created by circumstances beyond the control of national leaders; thus the leaders are not to be held responsible for it. In discussing the origins and impacts of a crisis, Edelman has argued:

It appears that the recurrence of crises is predictable because they flow from inequalities in economic and political power; but the burdens of almost all crises fall disproportionately on the poor, while the influential and the affluent often benefit from them. (1977, p. 44)

Various current crises are relevant to health and the aged. The most important of these can be summarized as follows:

1. A worldwide economic crisis has resulted in less "slack" in the economic system and in greater attention to fostering the conditions for renewed economic expansion.
2. Related to this economic crisis is a fiscal crisis of the state (as it attempts to underwrite the costs both of capital expansion and of those who are displaced by it), which has resulted in austerity policies threatening the welfare state.
3. Health care, which constitutes a major and increasing portion of government spending, is in jeopardy as a result of budget cutbacks, as are other areas of the welfare state.
4. Health services, equipment, facilities, and related products constitute a major industry, absorbing an increasing portion of the gross national product. However, this industry has operated in a manner that is not efficient from the point of view of capitalist accumulation.
5. The conjunction of these crisis factors will provide increasing pressure for significant cutbacks in health services and major changes in the structure of the health industry.

This is one view. Other commentators, taking the same conditions, may construe the crises differently. Those with sufficient power to do so may *declare* crises. And to such declarations, we must all, in some way, respond—whatever we believe the true, underlying crises to be.

The perceptions of crises and the designation of issues such as aging or health care as major national problems illustrate what Berger and Luckmann (1966) have called "the social construction of reality." A reality, once perceived, comes to exist because others believe and act as if it is real. Policy actions and social consequences flow from such definitions and perceptions, although they may represent only partial realities. Thus we have crises of health care and crises of aging.

The Social Construction of Reality: Health and Aging

The significance of the social construction of reality about old age and health is that it has provided the legitimating rationale or ideology that undergirds public policy in these areas. Three major constructions of reality are central to the political economy of health and aging in our society:

1. Aging tends to be characterized as a process of biological and physiological decline and decay.
2. Some elderly are seen as deserving, while others are seen as undeserving.
3. Old people and old age are seen as a problem to society. This problem is seen as both special and different and as one of crisis proportions. In this context, care for the elderly is seen to be a major contributing factor to the health care crisis said to be occurring.

Aging as a Biological Process

The first major perception, or construction of reality, is that aging is largely a physical and biological process of decrement and decline— the biomedical model of aging. As discussed in Chapter 1, the tendency to equate aging with disease is associated with the conceptualization of old age as a process of individual, biological, and/or

psychological decline. In addition to the potential negative consequences of linking aging and disease, the definition of aging as a
biomedical problem individualizes and medicalizes the aging process.
It obscures the understanding of how health in old age is related to
one's location in the social structure, including one's income, sex,
race, social class, and type of work, and to the economic conditions of
a free enterprise system.

One of the most important consequences of the biomedical
model has been the wholesale adoption of a medical services strategy,
which often has served as a substitute for inadequate policies in other
major areas such as income, employment, and housing. The dominant
perception has been that medical services, not income or employment, can address the primary problems of older persons. This
typification of aging as a physiological process treats the problems of
the aged, their illnesses, and their needs independently of social
causes. It posits solutions through the consumption of largely acute
care medical services. Far from draining the economy, this medically
dominated service strategy has, in fact, facilitated the economic
growth and expansion of human services technologies, industries, and
professions, and the biomedical research industry (see Chapter 4).
Thus the effect of current health policy, with its focus on Western
scientific medicine, has been to transform the multiple needs of the
aged into medical problems amenable to government-funded and
industry-developed interventions for specific economic markets
(Estes, 1979; 1982).

To summarize, several consequences may be associated with the
view of old age as an individual, and largely biological, process. First,
this view supports the idea that the origins of problems in old age
reside within the individual, thereby putting the blame on the victim.
It also diverts attention from problems generated by a society that
may reject or impoverish older people, or make them ill. This view
therefore strengthens the conservative notion that the best interventions and policies are those aimed at the individual level rather
than at collective social change. Second, this view lends support to the
continuing dominance of Western scientific medicine and to the
further development of the medical-industrial complex (Ehrenreich
and Ehrenreich, 1971; Relman, 1980). Third, the immense resource
investments required to support the aging enterprise and the medical-
industrial complex drain off needed societal resources from the
environment and from the adequate employment and income that are
essential to healthy aging. The contradiction is that the costs so
generated are used to blame the elderly for causing a crisis—for living
too long, for using too many health services, for not working long
enough, and for not saving enough.

The Deserving and the Undeserving

A second perception shaping public policy for the aged is that there are those who are deserving and those who are undeserving. Public policy for the elderly reflects these distinctions between different types of beneficiaries of public programs (Nelson, 1982; Estes, 1982). Those society deems to be deserving (the upper- and middle-income groups) receive benefits under uniform national policies (such as Medicare, Social Security, and tax credits) that are, in each instance, visible and universal. In contrast, those deemed undeserving (the lower-income groups) receive benefits under a myriad of highly variable state policies (such as Medicaid and SSI supplementation).

The notion of deservingness is not a new one; it dates back to seventeenth-century England and has been evident in the culture of the United States since the foundation of the Republic in the form of a Calvinistic doctrine (see Chapter 3). Identifying acceptable behavior and values, this doctrine exerted disciplinary control over the general populace by requiring conformance to normative standards of values such as hard work, thrift, and rugged individualism. In terms of public policy, an important aspect of deservingness is its utilization by the state to ration scarce resources. A society's idea of deservingness reflects and justifies commonly accepted beliefs and prejudices about who merits or deserves what and for what reasons. In this regard, lifelong discrimination patterns were often evident when decision makers applied this concept in the context of difficult policy choices and conflicting political demands among widely divergent social classes. Although the application of common principles of deservingness may vary according to state and regional differences and levels of government, the effect is the same throughout: deservingness as a criterion for resource allocation fosters competition between those groups seeking some public redress, placing whites against blacks, young against old, and rich against poor.

Although the notions of deservingness that were based on common prejudice have continued to be an underlying factor in public policy decisions, more identifiable categories of deservingness have emerged. In an early analysis of the welfare state, Titmuss (1965) identified three different types of public dependency: that derived from one's occupational status (earned rights), that derived from property ownership (vested rights), and that derived from disadvantaged minority group status, such as the poor without work or property (need-based entitlement). In U.S. society, those deemed the most deserving of public policy benefits have been the property owners with vested rights, followed by workers who had earned their benefit entitlements through years of union struggle and organization. The poor and disadvantaged have not been regarded as deserving of anything except where their needs arise out of an unalterable physical condition, such as age or disability, or a temporary limiting condition. The liberal mode of the early 1960s era was a basic movement to dramatically alter the commonly held subjective criteria of deservingness based on individual personality and behavior to more objective criteria of deservingness based on the impingement on individual opportunity created by the social institutions of discrimination, poverty, and social class.

Deservingness criteria may seem abstract but they are nevertheless extremely significant in revealing ideas that have become embedded in our social consciousness. These ideas shape our beliefs about what is possible and the political choices among competing and conflicting ends. Do old people deserve a greater share of the nation's health care resources because they are dependent, or do young people deserve more because they represent a national future investment? In answering such questions, bureaucratic agencies created by local, state, or federal government are called upon to exercise judgment in the allocation and distribution of health and social service resources. These political judgments are tempered by the interests of the dominant financial and economic institutions.

The Elderly and the Health Care Crisis

A third perception, which reflects a wider political and economic crisis, is that there is a health care crisis, and that the elderly are a significant part of the problem. As economic concerns have intensified and as health care costs have continued to rise two to three times the rate of inflation, policy makers, taxpayers, and patients who pay an increasing share of these costs have all declared a health care crisis. Such crises are, as we noted earlier, socially produced in the sense that they result from dominant societal perceptions. The attributes of the crisis are socially produced as well; that is, neither the crisis nor its primary attributes are objectively fixed or determined. Both emerge as a result of perception and definition.

The designated nature of this crisis has changed over the decades—most notably from a concern about access in the 1960s (precipitating the passage of Medicare and Medicaid) toward an overriding concern in the 1970s and 1980s with controlling rising health care costs. Along the way there has been a tension between those favoring the liberal approach of government regulation and planning and those favoring the conservative approach of a competitive market with deregulation. As currently defined and as represented in the media, the health crisis calls for cost control. Contemporary debate centers on how to achieve cost containment with the least harm to the different opponents' values (for example, free market or equity). The major constructions of reality about the health care crisis are that its solutions lie in one of two directions: competition or regulation.

Competition. Competition, in its most recent form, is based on the theory that if the free market is permitted to operate without either oppressive regulation or inappropriate subsidies for the purchase of health services, costs will be contained and a necessary level of services provided. The two key elements in the competitive approach are (1) increased cost sharing by individuals, in order that they be more responsive to price competition among providers, and (2) economic incentives for individuals to choose the health plan most suited to their needs and resources. Most advocates of price competition believe that there should be significant cost sharing by consumers at the time services (such as physician office visits, hospital admissions, or prescription drug purchases) are provided. Some of the advocates of price competition believe that all, or almost all, constraints should be lifted from professional medical advertising. Economist Milton Friedman would even eliminate all licensure requirements and would permit anyone who so desires to practice medicine or other healing arts.

The most widely advocated approach would require major reforms in the structure of the health service market, with a rapid expansion of prepaid memberships in health maintenance organizations and other organized systems of care. The costs for the purchase of such private third-party coverage would be shared more equally by employers and employees. (Employers now pay approximately 85 percent of private health insurance.) When workers and public beneficiaries share in the cost of health care, they will shop around for the most economical providers and insurance coverage (Enthoven, 1980). It is argued that insurers would contract only with cost-effective providers, giving providers incentives to deliver care at a lower cost. In essence, cost sharing is presumed to contain costs by inhibiting consumer use of services (Salmon, 1982).

In any case, the competitive model, as presented by economists, also signifies a change in the way we think about health care and the value society as a whole places on health and not merely a reorganization of personnel and services. Economists are fond of reiterating the observation, keenly felt by many these days, that resources are not unlimited. One elementary problem from an economic perspective, then, is how to ration scarce resources effectively in a world of seemingly unlimited human needs and wants. The precompetition strategy proposes to shift the responsibility for rationing of resources from the collective social level (that is, government) to that of the private individual level (that is, the consumer). Undoubtedly, this will affect some individuals more than others. Those who live on fixed incomes, the newly poor from eastern industrial regions, the near poor, and the poorest, who are all dependent on public programs, would be forced to ration their health care if they are required to seek such care with a voucher in hand. The cornerstone of the market system is best described as "a framework in which private decision-makers act in accordance with cues provided by the price system" (Blumstein, 1983, p. 351). If consumers become more price sensitive, so the theory goes, benefits and profits will simultaneously increase. While not a concern of the market system, equity considerations have been the major arguments given for public intervention in a market economy (Vladeck, 1981b; Blumstein, 1983). According to Vladeck (1981b), government intervention for the purpose of equitable distribution of resources is very important where more than 40 percent of an industry's revenue comes from public tax dollars.

Regulation. Regulation, another proposed solution to the health care crisis, is based on the theory that it is possible to rationally plan and coordinate the health care delivery system to achieve both cost control and equitable access. Such a solution theoretically would allow for the allocation of resources to different sectors of health care, as well as account for differences in patient needs, ability to pay, and availability of health care.

A number of regulatory mechanisms have characterized the health service sector, ranging from professional licensure (a state government function) to professional standards review organizations (PSRO's), which were federally mandated to review the appropriateness of hospital care provided to Medicare beneficiaries. Current regulations are most rigorous regarding the marketing of new drugs and devices. They are least restrictive with respect to new procedures developed and used by physicians, which go essentially unregulated. Regulation advocates favor several different approaches to the public regulation of hospital costs, nursing home costs, and physician costs. Some favor a public utility model of regulation, in which financing remains pluralistic (Medicare, Medicaid, private health insurance) but the price paid by all payers to all providers is regulated. Hospital costs may be controlled by limiting the hospital charges per day or per case. The diagnosis related group (DRG) prospective reimbursement policy adopted in 1983 by the Health Care Financing Administration for the Medicare program is based on costs per case. Others prefer a global budget for the hospital that limits the yearly increase. Global budgets may or may not relate to case mix and other factors, such as teaching.

In the United States, a growing number of states are moving toward all payer regulation of hospital costs, but none have yet moved to control physician fees paid by all payers. This provides an interesting contrast to the Reagan Administration's deregulation theme. The most effective control of health care costs among industrialized, Western nations has been achieved by Great Britain and Canada. In Great Britain, the entire system is centrally planned and budgeted, while in Canada, controls are achieved in a publicly funded system of national health insurance with global budgets for hospitals and negotiated fees for physicians.

The Class Basis of Sacrifice

If crises are declared in line with socially constructed perceptions and class interests, the recommended solutions are likewise so constructed. Public policy for the aged has already been molded according to such perceptions and interests in response to socially defined problems and crises. Insofar as the current era is one of particular crisis for which the chosen solution is austerity, or sacrifice, it is to be expected that such sacrifice will be apportioned according to the interests of those who define the crisis. In particular, there will be a class basis to the sacrifice.

Current old age policy in the United States reflects a two-tiered system of welfare with benefits distributed on the basis of legitimacy rather than on the basis of need (Tussing, 1971). Old age neither levels nor diminishes social class distinctions (Nelson, 1982; Estes, 1982; Crystal, 1982). It is the individual lifetime conditions and labor force participation established before retirement age that largely determine an older person's social class and economic resources (A. Walker, 1981). While we recognize class status to be much more complex than income status alone, which is itself an outcome of social policies, income represents a practical and available vehicle for examining class relationships related to policies for the aged.

The nonpoor elderly have resources that provide them access to public and private services largely without the necessity of government intervention. They also receive a disproportionately high share of the benefits from the largest federal programs for the aged, for example, Social Security, Medicare, and tax credits (Nelson, 1983). Those who are newly poor in old age are favored by social service policies. Because the newly poor are thought of as both deserving and deprived, services such as the Older Americans Act largely assist people in this downwardly mobile group to maintain their lifestyles, rather than providing crucial life-support income for the poor aged

(Nelson, 1982). The elderly who have been lifelong poor are assisted mostly through inadequate income-maintenance policies such as Supplemental Security Income (SSI), Medicaid (which is highly variable from state to state), food stamps, and the Social Security minimum benefit (now available only to current, not future beneficiaries). Table 6-1 shows the class basis of aging policies.

Deservingness in old age income policies is firmly rooted in the principle of differential rewards for differential achievements during a lifetime. For those individuals who, in the past, had been casually employed or who had low lifetime earnings covered by Social Security (mainly women and minorities), the minimum benefit guaranteed a basic monthly Social Security payment of $122. The successful Reagan Administration effort to eliminate the Social Security minimum benefit for all future beneficiaries (U.S. Public Law 97-35, 1981) illustrates the pressure to remove the "undeserving" aged from the receipt of Social Security benefits. Proponents of this policy change argue that those who require income support beyond what they have actually earned in the labor market should look to the means-tested Supplementary Security Income (SSI) program or to other state or local welfare programs for relief (U.S. House, Committee on Ways and Means, 1981).

Public policies such as Medicaid and SSI supplementation that affect the "undeserving," poorest aged have involved a significant measure of state discretion. Because the responsibility has rested with the states (Estes, 1982), both program eligibility and benefits for the poor have depended on the variable willingness and fiscal capacity of states to fund programs at the state or local level (Bovbjerg and Holahan, 1982). Not only have these state discretionary programs varied from state to state, they have also been more economically vulnerable than federal programs. Particularly in the current fiscal context of federal cutbacks in social programs, reduced taxation, high unemployment, and increased demands on the states, decisions about services for the poor are located precisely where pressures to control social expenses are greatest (and where the need to maintain the local economy also forces these governments to limit corporate taxes, while providing other economic incentives to business) (Friedland, Alford, and Piven, 1977; David and Kantor, 1981).

The effect of recent U.S. policy shifts slowing the growth in federal Medicaid costs and reducing other social spending has been to aggravate existing inequities in programs for the poor across the states (Estes and Newcomer, 1983). With the block grants created in the 1970s and 1980s easing the constraints of categorical funding and of federal requirements, there are pressures to reduce the programs that affect the most economically disadvantaged and vulnerable of all ages.

Table 6-1
Class Basis of Aging Policies

Policy area	Deserving elderly (1 federal policy) upper and middle income	Undeserving elderly (50 state variable policies) low income
Income		
Social Security (SS)	Highest payments to this group of wage earners; regressive taxation—no SS tax after $35,700 salary level	Payment structure hurts this group the most; minimum Social Security benefit eliminated for all future eligibles
private pensions tax policy	Individual Retirement Accounts (IRA); tax credits—Economic Recovery Tax Act of 1981	Little or no capacity to invest in private pensions
Supplemental Security Income (SSI)		Payment levels below poverty level; means-tested

Health		
Medicare program	Highest expenditures for this group; greater capacity to pay deductibles and copayments	Lower access to physicians and hospitals for blacks, other minorities, and the poor
Medicaid program[a]		Means-tested; approximately 50 percent of persons below poverty level not covered
private insurance	Greater capacity to purchase coverage	Little or no capacity to purchase coverage
Social services		
Social Services Block Grant (formerly Title XX of the Social Security Act)		No federally mandated priority to low-income eligibles
Older Americans Act[a]	Provides services most needed by middle class, such as information and referral, transportation	No federally mandated priority to low-income eligibles

[a]Variable state policies emerge primarily from state-federal programs in which states have much discretion over eligibility and scope of available services. State discretionary programs are highly vulnerable to swings in state fiscal capacity and political commitment to serve the needs of the poor.

An accurate assessment of the relation between public policy and social class in old age requires consideration of both direct and indirect government expenditures (Nelson, 1982). Direct expenditures include Social Security and Medicare while indirect expenditures involve tax policies. Tax savings constitute a federal expenditure because tax liability reductions represent federal revenue losses (U.S. Congressional Budget Office, 1982c). While direct federal expenditures benefit the poor and low-income groups, indirect federal expenditures favor the middle- and upper-income groups (Wilensky, 1982; Nelson, 1983). In 1982 alone, an estimated $43 billion in indirect federal expenditures were allocated largely to middle- and upper-income elderly (Nelson, 1983). These tax subsidies could pay for the estimated $12.7 billion in welfare expenditures for older people, since these tax savings for the well-off elderly constitute more than three times the elderly's share of program costs for Medicaid, SSI, Title XX, and food stamps combined. As Crystal (1982) has described it, public policy supports two highly unequal classes of elderly, both dependent on direct and indirect public aid. The gap between these "two worlds" of aging is widening—one is comfortable and the other is miserable and destitute. Health status is inequitably distributed between the two worlds as well, with the poorer one plagued by chronic illness and the richer one characterized by good health.

The class bias of federal policy shifts, tax cuts, and budget cuts since 1981 has been extensively documented (Palmer and Sawhill, 1982; U.S. Senate Special Committee on Aging, 1982a; Havemann, 1982; McIntyre and Tipps, 1983). Simply stated, the tax cuts significantly benefit households with annual incomes over $80,000, augmenting their income by more than $55 billion. In contrast, households with incomes under $10,000 will actually lose $17 billion in income between 1983 and 1985 (Greenstein and Bickerman, 1983). When tax bills are adjusted for inflation, real tax bills will rise 22 percent between 1980 and 1984 for families earning less than $10,000. Only families earning more than $30,000 will get real tax breaks, and only the top 5 percent of taxpayers (those earning over $100,000) will enjoy significant cuts (McIntyre and Tipps, 1983, p. 22). Figure 6-1 gives the average tax changes of the Reagan/Kemp-Roth rate cuts.

The opposite effects hold for budget cuts. The Congressional Budget Office reported that by 1985, 45 percent of the benefit reductions will be taken from the households in the under $10,000 annual income category; 25 percent will fall on households in the $10,000 to $20,000 category. Households with $80,000 and up in annual income will receive less than 1 percent of the cuts (U.S. Congressional Budget Office, 1982a; 1982b). The highly respected

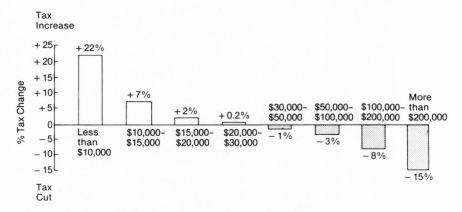

Figure 6-1. Average Percent Tax Changes from the Reagan/Kemp-Roth Rate Cuts by Income Class, 1982–1984 (after offsetting tax increases from inflation and higher Social Security taxes)

Source: From *Inequality and Decline: How the Reagan Tax Policies Are Affecting the American Taxpayer and the Economy*. By Robert S. McIntyre and Dean C. Tipps. Copyright © 1983 Center on Budget and Policy Priorities.

National Journal (Havemann, 1982) has reported that the poorest 20 percent of the population will have only 4.2 percent of the national income after federal taxes, while the richest 20 percent will have 43 percent. Even more impressive is the fact that, before the administration's tax and expenditure cuts and shifts were made, "the U.S. already had the most unequal income distribution of any Western industrialized country except France" (Greenstein and Bickerman, 1983, p. 6, from Thurow, 1981).

Because female and minority households have lower incomes, they are receiving a disproportionately large share of benefit cuts and a disproportionately small share of the benefits of tax reductions. Thus the wealth redistribution has accelerated the shift of resources from females to males and from minorities to whites in the United States (Greenstein and Bickerman, 1983; Coalition, 1983). Storey (1983) has documented that among the elderly those with annual household incomes below $5,000 have been affected most by the recent benefit reductions in food stamps, energy assistance, subsidized housing, minimum Social Security benefits, Medicaid, Comprehensive Employment and Training Act (CETA) opportunities, transit subsidies, and social services. Because of the substantially higher percentage of elderly who are female and their substantially lower incomes (72 percent of the elderly poor are female, and nearly half of all minority older women are poor), both the benefit cuts and tax reductions disadvantage older women and minorities.

The Class Bias in Health Policy

The inequities in Medicare benefits reported for low-income and minority elderly are significant in view of the direct relationship between health and income discussed in Chapter 5. Recent policy changes have exacerbated these inequities, particularly for the near-poor elderly. Escalating health care costs and budget cuts totaling nearly $18 billion by the end of 1985 have raised the proportion of costs shouldered by Medicare recipients. The result is increased economic hardship for those least able to afford it. Health care costs exceeded $1,100 in per capita out-of-pocket costs in 1981 and are expected to amount to $1,546 in 1983 (U.S. Senate, Special Committee on Aging, 1983, p. 394). These costs are sobering in view of the fact that the median income for the elderly in 1980 was $4,226 (Storey, 1983).

Budget reductions are being accomplished in part by increasing the proportion of costs shouldered by Medicare recipients. Deductibles (the base amount one pays before care becomes covered) and copayments (the proportion of total charges payable by beneficiaries) have both increased dramatically in the past two years. The Part A deductible increased 27 percent between 1981 and 1982 (from $204 to $260), more than double the historical increase. The Part B deductible for 1982 rose 25 percent (from $60 to $75). The Part A levels for both hospital and skilled nursing facility care also were increased, and reimbursement levels to radiologists and pathologists were reduced from 100 percent, exposing the beneficiary to new cost-sharing levels of 20 percent for these services. Proposals for increased cost sharing would add copayments (a percentage of the hospital deductible) for a certain number of days of hospital care. The added out-of-pocket costs for the 20 percent of elderly hospitalized each year would be significant—projected for 1983 at $268 at least, and $301 for those 80 and older (U.S. Senate Special Committee on Aging, 1983b). Additional cost-sharing proposals include modifying the rate of increase in the Part B physician premium and increasing its deductible, as well as establishing a voluntary voucher proposal.

When applied equally to all Medicare beneficiaries, the differential impact of these flat rate proposals becomes clear. If expressed as a percentage of average income, the differences in medical expenditures among income groups is striking (see Figure 6-2). The Congres-

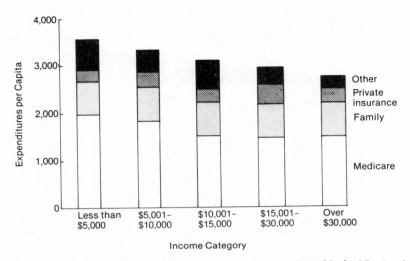

Figure 6-2. Annual Per Capita Medical Expenditures for Elderly Noninstitutionalized Medicare Enrollees, by Source of Payment and Income (in 1984 dollars)

Note: The amounts shown here indicate payments for health care services. Consequently, the private insurance category consists of payments to providers from insurance companies and does not include premiums paid to insurance companies.

Source: National Medical Care Expenditure Survey. Congressional Budget Office. *Changing the Structure of Medicare Benefits: Issues and Options*. Washington, D.C.: Government Printing Office, March 1983, Figure 3.

sional Budget Office projects that

> by 1984 noninstitutionalized persons with household incomes under $5,000 will have medical expenditures totalling 97 percent of their $3,659 average income, 18 percent of which they must pay out-of-pocket. Those in the highest income category are expected to have expenditures representing less than 5 percent of their projected average income of $58,306 and will pay just over 1 percent out-of-pocket (U.S. CBO, 1983, p. 21)

The increases in copayments and deductibles are expected to increase the out-of-pocket payments for the aged and to: (1) increase the number of aged who cannot afford to purchase Part B Medicare coverage of physician services, (2) increase the price of supplemental insurance so that many of the aged will not be able to purchase it, and (3) increase the number of physicians who refuse assignment, thus further increasing costs and inaccessibility to the aged. The small increase in coverage for catastrophic insurance is not expected to

Table 6-2

Impact of Different Out-of-Pocket Health Care Expenditures on the Mean Income of Various Elderly Subgroups, 1981

1981 Per capita out-of-pocket health expenditures of the elderly:	$1,154
percent of mean income for all older persons	13%
percent of mean income for older women	17%
percent of mean income for older blacks	23%
percent of mean income for older black women	27%
1981 Per capita out-of-pocket health expenditures, less nursing home costs, for the noninstitutionalized elderly population:	$834[a]
percent of mean income for all older persons	9.5%
percent of mean income for older women	12.5%
percent of mean income for older blacks	16.5%
percent of mean income for older black women	19.8%

[a]Assumes noninstitutionalized elderly population equals 95 percent of total elderly population.
Source: New York State Office for the Aging. Medicare: Analysis and Recommendations for Reform. Albany, New York: September 1983, p. 16.

offset the increased costs to the elderly for Medicare (Harrington, 1983).

Table 6-2 further illustrates the inequities that these policy shifts are augmenting. Per capita out-of-pocket health care expenses are disproportionately borne by older blacks and women over other elderly. A recent review of this issue as it affects women is illustrative:

> After income, access to affordable health care is a major concern of the elderly. Budget cuts proposed for Medicare [for 1984] will hit women hard. While men have higher rates of fatal diseases and more days of hospital care, women have more long-term chronic diseases and longer length of stay in hospitals. (Length of stay is not unrelated to the fact that women make up 80 percent of the elderly who live alone, and for whom a return from the hospital requires a greater capacity for self-care.) On average, the elderly have hospital stays of eleven days, and only two percent of Medicare beneficiaries will benefit from the proposed catastrophic coverage which begins on the 61st day in the hospital. (Leadership Council of Aging Organizations, 1983, pp. 41–42)

Because minorities and other low-income elderly are disproportionately in poor health (see Chapter 5), the increased Medicare cost sharing is not the only policy change to affect these disadvantaged elderly. Those on Social Security and those on Supplemental Security

Income have lost income from delayed cost-of-living increases. (Some delays were federally engineered and some resulted from state actions freezing or reducing state SSI supplementation and/or cost-of-living increases for SSI recipients.) Particularly serious are Medicaid cutbacks imposed at both federal and state levels. In 1981, federal Medicaid costs were reduced by nearly $1 billion a year. Further federal cuts were added in 1982, and the states are themselves invoking major cost containment strategies to reduce Medicaid costs. Medicaid studies indicate that the strategies adopted by most states between 1979 and 1982 were designed to reduce directly the number of Aid to Families with Dependent Children clients and to reduce indirectly those who were "medically needy." This hurt those low-income elderly who were not income-eligible for SSI, but who had previously been considered Medicaid-eligible because of near-poverty income and high medical costs. States have tightened the eligibility floor (Newcomer and Harrington, 1983). Since two-thirds of the 22 million people eligible for Medicaid and 73 percent of SSI elderly are female, these Medicaid cuts will have a disproportionately negative impact on women:

> Mandatory co-payments, even for emergency care, are intended to discourage unnecessary health expenditures. Persons with chronic illnesses, which older women tend to have, will pay the most, with no limit on the total amounts each Medicaid recipient would be required to pay. Even more, there is no evidence that the elderly have misused either Medicare or Medicaid and, thus, need to be made more "cost conscious" through co-payments and deductibles. On average, older women are currently spending *one-third* of their median annual income for health care, and hardly need reminders about what it costs. What such proposals will do is discourage use of care until health problems become acute (and expensive), or leave older women with even less income for other necessities. (Leadership Council of Aging Organizations, 1983, p. 42)

Most states have placed limitations on the amount, duration, and scope of services. Many of the limitations have direct negative effects on the elderly such as copayments for drugs and restrictions on eyeglasses and dentures. Since 1982, states have been permitted to impose cost sharing on optional services for Medicaid recipients. New proposals are to *require* Medicaid cost sharing for physician, clinic, and hospital services (both outpatient and inpatient) and to extend federal Medicaid reductions beyond 1984 (Newcomer and Harrington, 1983).

Several factors make these program cuts particularly difficult for minority elderly. For example, blacks have twice the rate of disablement from chronic illness that whites do. Elderly black men and black women are significantly poorer. Thirty percent of Medicaid recipients are black. Thirty-two percent and 43 percent of black men and women, respectively, are in poverty, compared with only 8 percent of elderly white males and 16 percent of elderly white females. In perhaps the most important indicator of access, blacks are much less likely to hold supplemental insurance (Medigap) to cover their health expenses than are whites (73 percent of whites compared to 32 percent of blacks) (Leadership Council of Aging Organizations, 1983).

Consequences of Public Policy

In the United States we have paid a heavy price for our deep-rooted commitment to the market ideology, to individualism, and to competition. Among Western industrialized nations, the United States is the most generous with respect to benefits to corporations and to those with high income. Disproportionate costs are borne by working people, particularly the working poor. Magaziner and Reich (1982) have shown, that compared to European countries, the United States:

- has smaller social welfare spending as a percentage of the gross national product
- is the only country without some form of national health insurance
- has a lower life expectancy at birth than most of these other countries
- has a higher infant mortality rate than most
- has had higher average unemployment over the past twenty years than all of these other countries except Canada
- covers a smaller proportion of the unemployed with unemployment insurance and pays lower unemployment benefits (as a percentage of prior wages)
- has a less equal distribution of income (that is, more of a gap between the incomes of the top and bottom of the society) than all of these countries except France
- has higher pollution levels (and less strict environmental controls) than most of these other countries

Although there is no simple causal explanation for the poor health status of the United States compared to its counterparts in the Western industrial world and even some Third World nations, it is difficult to disassociate these effects from beliefs, attitudes, ideologies, and public policies. The potential consequences of the growing acceptance of the competitive ideology in health are profound, for this acceptance signals support for the notion that the individual, not society or other factors beyond the control of the individual, is to blame for health status and health costs.

Ideology is a major factor affecting the environment in which the elderly receive and physicians provide health care. In recent years, two themes have been repeated over and over again: (1) government is too big and too intrusive, and (2) social problems, such as health care costs, access, and quality, are best solved by the market influences and not by government intervention. These two ideological themes, combined with fiscal realities, have led many political leaders to talk about an era of austerity and an era of limits, to stress cost-effectiveness in medical care, and to propose policies to reduce regulation and stimulate price competition (Lee, 1983).

This ideological shift has led to the notion that the intrusion of large corporations into health care—particularly in the ownership of hospitals, nursing homes, dialysis centers, surgicenters, clinical laboratories, and other large and small providers—is for the good. In 1981, profit-making hospital chains owned or managed hospitals with 121,745 beds, a 68 percent increase over their bed total five years earlier. In the same year, more than 300 hospitals, with 43,000 beds, were owned by one company, the Hospital Corporation of America (Starr, 1982). The big proprietary firms own or manage 12 percent of the nation's hospitals and 8 percent of the hospital beds. These figures are expected to more than double in the next decade (see Chapter 4). The gross patient revenue of investor-owned hospitals reached almost $10 billion in 1980. Corporations are also buying or opening freestanding ambulatory surgical centers, freestanding emergency/primary care centers, dialysis centers, and dental offices. Ideology explains how, despite little "evidence to suggest that the for-profit companies achieve any savings over non-profits" (Starr, 1982, p. 433), conservative rhetoric continues to support public policies aimed at reducing government regulation through the initiation of competitive strategies.

The Medicare voucher is one particularly important competitive health strategy that has surfaced politically and that would vitally affect the elderly. Elderly individuals would be given the amount of the average annual per capita Medicare cost (adjusted for age, sex, disability, and geography) to purchase private health insurance or to enroll in prepaid health plans. Under some proposals, if premiums for the private plans were less than the Medicare per capita costs, cash rebates would be provided to the elderly. If costs or services needed were to exceed those covered in the purchased insurance plan, the elderly would incur the added costs. The incentive for the elderly would be to purchase the lowest cost insurance and probably to underinsure themselves, thereby ultimately paying more out of their own income.

There are serious risks that the voucher program may not reduce, but might actually *increase*, health costs inasmuch as: "Medicare expenditures are not spread evenly over the elderly, but are concentrated on a few, very sick individuals" (Davis, 1982, p. 29) whose costs average over $7,000 per year (8.8 percent of enrollees). As Davis notes, 76.6 percent of Medicare enrollees average $62 a year in medical care costs. Giving them all a voucher for the estimated $2,200 annual per capita cost in fiscal year 1984 to purchase health insurance would undoubtedly be very costly to the public treasury. Furthermore, there is concern that the private plans can be expected to market to the healthier elderly in order to reduce costs and increase profits, leaving the sickest and poorest elderly uninsured by the private plans—and thus necessitating their public coverage through Medicare. If successfully enacted, the Medicare voucher plan would accelerate the corporatization of health care for the elderly, as well as profits for private industry, and all at public expense.

The New Class War in Health

Medicine and health now represent a battleground in which a "new class war" (Piven and Cloward, 1982) is being fought. The combination of social program cuts, inflation reduction, and unemployment-generating policies has enlarged the bargaining power of employers and weakened that of workers. This has exacted severe restrictive pressures on both wages and benefits and created expansionary boosts for profits. In the health arena, the conflicts appear to be shaping up not only between the mass of health consumers and the controllers of health care institutions but also within the provider class between the private sector interests in entrepreneurial medicine (for example, private fee-for-service medical practitioners) and corporate medical interests over the financing of the health sector (Navarro, 1975b).

Myles's (1984) thoughts on the issue are cogent. Contrasting the liberal democratic state with the capitalist economy, he has pointed out the very different principles guiding these two forms of social organization. From the liberal democratic polity arose the notion of "rights" based on citizenship rather than ownership, property, and economic power. Health policy in the United States has reflected this underlying tension of values over the past century. One value has promoted the concept of health care as a merit good, in other words, as a good in and of itself and as an entitlement based on the rights of citizenship. This value evolved over the years in the context of the labor struggle for greater equality, representation, and protection in the democratic state. In contrast, the other value of health has promoted the concept of health care as a market good, in other words, as a good that can be transformed into a commodity for sale and profit in the medical care market. The principle of health care as a merit good arose from the liberal democratic polity, whereas the principle of health care as a market good arose from the basic values of the capitalist economic system. The major question that Myles (1984) raises is whether there is an inherent incompatibility between the requisites of a capitalist economy and a democracy. The duality and contradiction in values surrounding health policy are reflected in ongoing debate about the crisis in health care and its solutions.

These conflicts and contradictions are occurring in an environment of fiscal and economic crises. Although these crises involve real political and economic problems based on the world economic system, they will likely continue to be defined in terms of a narrower politics, particularly in terms of the need to cut social spending. Those advocating social spending will be hard pressed to defend it in such an environment, especially if the present economic downturn continues or reappears. Expansion of social spending, such as that seen in the 1960s, is unlikely to reappear. This means that advocates for services for the elderly will be fighting mostly defensive battles, often at best giving up on some benefits in order to save others.

What are the likely consequences of the dramatic changes in public policies designed to contain health care costs? What will be the effects of the cutbacks in programs for the poor, the growing emphasis on price competition and the marketplace, and, finally, the rapid expansion of corporate medicine? In the short run, we foresee two major developments:

- Reduced demand for medical care is likely because of the loss of private health insurance by the unemployed, tighter restrictions on Medicaid eligibility, and the shift in Medicare to greater consumer cost sharing. This will further disadvantage the elderly (particularly women and minorities), pregnant women, infants, and children because of reduced access to necessary medical care.
- Increased price competition is likely to accelerate the commodification of health.

In the longer term, a number of conflicts will arise, particularly if present trends in health care and public policy continue (Starr, 1982). Within the medical establishment itself, there is likely to be increased conflict between practicing physicians and hospital management (Alford, 1976). As physicians try to gain more control over a larger share of the health care dollar through such mechanisms as multi-specialty group practice and health maintenance organizations, hospitals will attempt to expand into areas traditionally controlled by physicians, such as ambulatory care. Within corporate medicine there is likely to be growing conflict between the nonprofit sector and the for-profit corporations that are now expanding so rapidly. With increased industry concentration, there are likely to be conflicts between local needs, as defined by the communities, local public agencies, and consumers, and the direction of health care corporations that are either regional or national in their scope. Just as General Motors thinks in terms of its profits and corporate needs rather than of the needs of a community when it closes a plant, so may profit and corporate interests in the field of health conflict with community needs and interests. According to Starr:

> This turn of events is the fruit of a history of accommodating professional and institutional interests, failing to exercise public control over public programs, then adopting piecemeal regulation to control inflationary consequences and, as a final resort, cutting back programs and turning them back to the private sector. (1982, p. 449)

Overview

In summary, various factors will result in a significantly more stratified medical care system that is characterized by increased inequalities in access to health care. These factors include:

· increasing emphasis on price competition to solve the problems of cost, access, and quality health care
· shifting of the burden of financial responsibility from the federal to state governments and from the state to local governments and to individuals
· increasing fragmentation of third-party reimbursement policies, aimed at controlling costs rather than assuring equity, access, or quality
· the fact that the government is increasingly acting as simply another interest group (Lowi, 1969; 1971) in defending industry interests in health

In contrast with these developments, the President's Commission on Ethical Problems in Medicine and Biomedical and Behavioral Research has clearly reaffirmed the national health goal of the 1960s as continuing to provide the correct direction for federal health policies in the 1980s.

> The Commission concludes that society has an ethical obligation to ensure equitable access to health care for all. This obligation rests on the special importance of health care: its role in relieving suffering, prevent-

ing premature death, restoring functioning, increasing opportunity, providing information about an individual's condition and giving evidence of mutual empathy and compassion. Furthermore, although life style and the environment can affect health status, differences in the need for health care are for the most part undeserved and not within an individual's control. (U.S. President's Commission, 1983, p. 4)

The commission, while recognizing the necessity of sharing the burden of health care costs between the individual and society, emphasized that the ultimate responsibility for ensuring that society's obligation is met rests with the federal government. We concur.

References

Abbott, J. "Socioeconomic Characteristics of the Elderly: Some Black-White Differences." *Social Security*, 40, No. 7 (July 1977), 16–42.

Achenbaum, W. A. *Old Age in the New Land: The American Experience Since 1970.* Baltimore: Johns Hopkins University Press, 1978.

_____. *Shades of Gray: Old Age, American Values, and Federal Policies Since 1920.* Boston: Little, Brown, 1983.

Aday, L. A., and R. M. Andersen. "Equity of Access to Medical Care: A Conceptual and Empirical Overview." *Medical Care*, 19, No. 12, Supplement (December 1981), 4–27.

Alford, R. *Health Care Politics*. Chicago: University of Chicago Press, 1976.

Altmeyer, A. J. *The Formative Years of Social Security*. Madison, Wis.: University of Wisconsin Press, 1966.

Amin, S., et al., eds. *Dynamics of Global Crises*. New York: Monthly Review, 1982.

Andreano, R. L., and B. A. Weisbrod. *American Health Policy: Perspectives and Choices*. Chicago: Rand McNally, 1974.

Antonovsky, A. "Social Class, Life Expectancy and Overall Mortality." *Milbank Memorial Fund Quarterly*, 45, No. 2, Pt. 1 (1967), 31–73.

Arluke, A., and J. Peterson. "Accidental Medicalization of Old Age and Its Social Control Implications." In *Dimensions: Aging, Culture, and Health*, edited by C. L. Frye. Brooklyn, N.Y.: J. F. Bergen, 1981.

Arrow, K. J. "Uncertainty and the Welfare Economics of Medical Care." *The American Economic Review*, 58, No. 5 (December 1963), 941–973.

Atchley, R. C. "Social Class and Aging." *Generations: Journal of the Western Gerontological Society*, 6, No. 2 (Winter 1981), 16–17.

Bachrach, P. *The Theory of Democratic Elitism: A Critique*. Boston: Little, Brown, 1967.

Ball, R. M. "Rethinking National Policy on Health Care for the Elderly," In

The Geriatric Imperative, edited by A. R. Somers and D. R. Fabian, New York: Appleton-Century-Crofts, 1981.

Becker, H. S. *Outsiders*. New York: Free Press of Glencoe, 1963.

Berger, P., and T. Luckmann. *The Social Construction of Reality*. New York: Doubleday, 1966.

Berliner, H. S. "Emerging Ideologies in Medicine." *The Review of Radical Political Economics*, 9, No. 1 (Spring 1977), 116–123.

Binstock, R. H. "The Aged as Scapegoat." Kent Award Lecture presented at the annual meeting of the Gerontological Society of America, November 22, 1982, Boston.

Birren, J. E. *The Psychology of Aging*. Englewood Cliffs, N.J.: Prentice-Hall, 1964.

Block, M. R. "Exiled Americans: The Plight of Indian Aged in the United States." In *Ethnicity and Aging*, edited by D. E. Gelfand and A. J. Kutzik. New York: Springer, 1979.

Blum, H. L. "A National Health Policy." Paper presented at Conference on National Health Policy Issues, February 12–13, 1976, San Francisco.

Blumstein, J. F. "Rationing Medical Resources: A Constitutional, Legal, and Policy Analysis." In *Security Access to Health Care: The Ethical Implications of Differences in the Availability of Health Services*, Vol. 3. Washington, D.C.: President's Commission for the Study of Ethical Problems in Medicine and Biomedical and Behavioral Research, 1983.

Bovbjerg, R. R., and J. Holahan. *Medicaid in the Reagan Era*. Washington, D.C.: Urban Institute, 1982.

Bowen, W., and T. A. Finegan. *The Economics of Labor Force Participation*. Princeton, N.J.: Princeton University Press, 1969.

Brenner, M. H. *Mental Illness and the Economy*. Cambridge, Mass.: Harvard University Press, 1973.

———. "Effects of National Economic Trends on Utilization of General Hospitals." Paper presented at the annual meeting of the American Public Health Association, November 16–20, 1975a, Chicago.

———. "Trends in Alcohol Consumption and Associated Illnesses." *American Journal of Public Health*, 65, No. 12 (December 1975b), 1279–1292.

———. "Reply to Mr. Eyer." *International Journal of Health Services*, 6, No. 1 (1976), 149–155.

Brody, E. M. "'Women in the Middle' and Family Help to Older People." *Gerontologist*, 21, No. 5 (October 1981), 471–480.

Brotman, H. B. *Every Ninth American*. Washington, D.C.: U.S. Government Printing Office, 1982.

Brown, E. R. *Rockefeller Medicine Men: Medicine and Capitalism in America*. Berkeley, Calif.: University of California Press, 1979.

———. "Medicare and Medicaid: Band-aids for the Old and Poor." Unpublished manuscript, School of Public Health, University of California, Los Angeles, 1982.

Bruhn, J. G. "An Ecological Perspective of Aging." *The Gerontologist*, 11, No. 4, Pt. 1 (Winter 1971), 318–321.

Buchanan, R. J. "The Financial Status of the New Medical-Industrial Complex." *Inquiry*, 19 (Winter 1982), 308–316.

118   References

Burke, V. J., and V. Burke. "Supplemental Security Income." In *The Aging in Politics*, edited by R. B. Hudson. Springfield, Ill.: Charles C. Thomas, 1981.

Butler, L. H., and P. W. Newacheck. "Health and Social Factors Affecting Long-Term Care Policy." In *Policy Options in Long-Term Care*, edited by J. Meltzer, F. Farrow, and H. Richman. Chicago: University of Chicago Press, 1981.

Butler, L. H., P. W. Newacheck, et al. "Low Income and Illness: An Analysis of National Health Policy and the Poor." Health Policy Program Working Paper. San Francisco: University of California Press, 1981.

Butler, R. N., and M. I. Lewis. *Aging and Mental Health*, 3rd ed. St. Louis, Mo.: Mosby, 1982.

Cain, G. G., and H. Watts. "Toward a Summary and Synthesis of the Evidence." In *Income Maintenance and Labor Supply*, edited by G. G. Cain and H. Watts. New York: Academic, 1973.

Calhoun, R. B. *In Search of the New Old*. New York: Elsevier, 1978.

Cassel, J. "Psychosocial Processes and 'Stress': Theoretical Formulation." *International Journal of Health Services*, 4, No. 3 (1974), 471–482.

Castells, M. *The Economic Crisis and American Society*. Princeton, N.J.: Princeton University Press, 1980.

_____. *City, Class and Power*. New York: St. Martin's, 1982.

Cater, D., and P. R. Lee, eds. *Politics of Health*. New York: Medcom, 1972.

Clark, R. L., and J. L. Spengler. *The Economics of Individual and Population Aging*. London: Cambridge University Press, 1980.

Clarke, G. J. "In Defense of Deinstitutionalization." *Milbank Memorial Fund Quarterly/Health and Society*, 57, No. 4 (1979) 461–479.

Coalition on Women and the Budget. *Inequality of Sacrifice: The Impact of the Reagan Budget on Women*. Washington, D.C.: National Women's Law Center, 1983.

Collins, R. "Comparative Approach to Political Sociology." In *State and Society*, edited by R. Bendix et al. Boston: Little, Brown, 1968.

Comfort, A. *A Good Age*. New York: Crown, 1976.

Committee for Economic Development (CED). "Building a National Health-Care System." New York: CED, 1973.

Connolly, W. E. *The Bias of Pluralism*. New York: Atherton, 1969.

Conrad, P., and R. Kern, eds. *The Sociology of Health and Illness: Critical Perspectives*. New York: St. Martin's, 1981.

Conrad, P., and J. W. Schneider. *Deviance and Medicalization: From Badness to Sickness*. St. Louis, Mo.: Mosby, 1980.

Cooley, C. H. *Human Nature and the Social Order*. New York: Schocken, 1964.

Cooper, J. W. "Pharmacology: Drug Related Problems and the Elderly." In *Eldercare: A Practical Guide to Clinical Geriatrics*, edited by M. O'Hara-Devereaux, L. H. Andrus, and C. D. Scott. New York: Grune and Stratton, 1981.

Crystal, S. *America's Old Age Crisis*. New York: Basic, 1982.

Cumming, E., and W. E. Henry. *Growing Old: The Process of Disengagement*. New York: Basic, 1961.

Dahl, R. A. *A Preface to the Democratic Theory*. Chicago: University of Chicago Press, 1956.

David, S. M., and P. Kantor. "Urban Policy in the Federal Systems: A Reconceptualization of Federalism." Paper presented at the annual meeting of the American Political Science Association, September 25, 1981, New York.

Davidson, S. M., and T. R. Marmor. *The Cost of Living Longer*. Lexington, Mass.: Heath, 1980.

Davis, K. "Equal Treatment and Unequal Benefits: The Medicare Program." *Milbank Memorial Fund Quarterly/Health and Society*, 53, No. 4 (1975), 449–488.

———. "Medicaid Payments and Utilization of Medical Services by the Poor." *Inquiry*, 13, No. 2 (June 1976), 122–135.

———. "Long Term Care for the Elderly: The Challenge to the States." Paper presented to the Health Care Financing Administration Conference on Long Term Care and the Elderly, September 9, 1981, Atlanta, Georgia.

———. "Medicare Reconsidered." Paper presented for the Duke University Medical Center Seventh Private Sector Conference on the Financial Support of Health Care of the Elderly and the Indigent, March 14–16, 1982, Durham, N.C.

———. "Health Implications of Aging in America." Unpublished manuscript, Johns Hopkins University, Baltimore, 1983.

Davis, K., and C. Schoen. *Health and the War on Poverty: A Ten Year Approach*. Washington, D.C.: Brookings Institution, 1978.

Derthick, M. *Policy-Making for Social Security*. Washington, D.C.: Brookings Institution, 1979.

Douglas, P. H. *Social Security in the United States*. New York: Whittlesey, 1936.

Dowd, J. J. "Aging as Exchange: A Preface to Theory." *Journal of Gerontology*, 30, No. 5 (1975), 584–594.

———. *Stratification Among the Aged*. Monterey, Calif.: Brooks/Cole, 1980.

Doyal, L. *The Political Economy of Health*. Boston: South End, 1979.

Duffy, M., E. Barrington, J. M. Flanagan, and L. Olson. *Inflation and the Elderly*. Lexington, Mass.: Data Resources, Inc., 1980.

Dunham, A. B., and T. R. Marmor. "Federal Policy and Health: Recent Trends and Differing Perspectives." In *Nationalizing Government: Public Policies in America*, edited by T. J. Lowi and A. Stone. Beverly Hills, Calif.: Sage, 1978.

Dunlop, B. D. *The Growth of Nursing Home Care*. Lexington, Mass.: Heath, 1979.

Edelman, M. *The Symbolic Uses of Politics*. Urbana, Ill.: University of Illinois Press, 1964.

———. *Politics as Symbolic Action*. Chicago: Markham, 1971.

———. *Political Language: Words That Succeed and Policies That Fail*. New York: Academic Press, 1977.

Edwards, C. C. "The Federal Involvement in Health." *New England Journal of Medicine*, 292 (13 March 1975), 559–562.

Ehrenreich, B., and J. Ehrenreich. *The American Health Empire: Power, Profits and Politic Empire*. New York: Vintage, 1971.

_____. "Health Care and Social Control." *Social Policy*, 5, No. 2 (1974), 26–40.

_____. "The Professional-Managerial Class." In *Between Labor and Capital*, edited by P. Walker. Boston: South End, 1979.

Ehrenreich, J. "Toward a Healing Society." *Social Policy*, 8, No. 5 (March-April 1978), 16–21.

Emrich, J. S. "The Capital Formation Process: An Institutional Perspective." In *Health Capital Issues*, DHEW Publication No. HRA 81-14531. Washington, D.C.: U. S. Department of Health and Human Services, 1980.

Enthoven, A. C. *Health Plan: The Only Solution to the Soaring Cost of Medical Care*. Reading, Mass.: Addison-Wesley, 1980.

Epstein, A. *Insecurity: A Challenge to America*. New York: Harrison Smith and Haas, 1936.

Estes, C. L. *The Aging Enterprise*. San Francisco: Jossey-Bass, 1979.

_____. "Austerity and Aging in the United States: 1980 and Beyond." *International Journal of Health Services*, 12, No. 4 (November 1982), 573–584.

_____. "Social Security: The Social Construction of a Crisis." *Milbank Memorial Fund Quarterly/Health and Society*, 61, No. 3 (1983), 445–461.

Estes, C. L., and L. Gerard. "Governmental Responsibility: Issues of Reform and Federalism." In *Fiscal Austerity and Aging*, by C. L. Estes and R. J. Newcomer, eds. Beverly Hills, Calif.: Sage, 1983.

Estes, C. L., L. Gerard, and A. Clark. "Women and the Economics of Aging." *International Journal of Health Services*, 14, No. 1 (1984), 55–68.

Estes, C. L., and C. Harrington. "Fiscal Crisis, Deinstitutionalization and the Elderly." *American Behavioral Scientist*, 24, No. 6 (July/August 1981), 811–826.

Estes, C. L., P. R. Lee, C. Harrington, et al. *Long-Term Care for California's Elderly: Policies to Deal with a Costly Dilemma*, California Policy Seminar Monograph No. 10. Berkeley, Calif.: Institute for Governmental Studies, University of California, 1981.

Estes, C. L., and R. J. Newcomer, eds. *Fiscal Austerity and Aging*. Beverly Hills, Calif.: Sage, 1983.

Estes, C. L., J. Swan, and L. Gerard. "Dominant and Competing Paradigms in Gerontology: Toward a Political Economy of Ageing." *Ageing and Society*, 2, Pt. 2 (July 1982), 151–164.

Evans, L., and J. Williamson. "Social Security and Social Control." *Generations: Journal of the Western Gerontological Society*, 6, No. 2 (Winter 1981), 18–20.

Eve, S. B., and H. J. Friedsam. "Use of Tranquilizers and Sleeping Pills Among Older Texans." In *Drugs, Alcohol and Aging*, edited by D. M. Petersen and F. J. Whittington. Dubuque, Iowa: Kendall/Hunt, 1982.

Eyer, J. "Rejoinder to Dr. Brenner." *International Journal of Health Services*, 6, No. 1 (1976a), 157–168.

_____. "Review of Mental Illness and the Economy." *International Journal of Health Services*, 6, No. 1 (1976b), 139–148.

Falk, I. S. "Medical Care: Its Social and Organizational Aspects." *New England Journal of Medicine*, 270, No. 1 (2 January 1964), 22–28.

Feder, J. M. "Medicare Implementation and the Policy Process." *Journal of Health Politics, Policy and Law*, 2, No. 2 (Summer 1977), 173–189.

Feldstein, P. J. *Health Associations and the Demand for Legislation: The Political Economy of Health*. Cambridge, Mass.: Ballinger, 1977.

Filner, B., and W. F. Williams. "Health Promotion for the Elderly." In *The Geriatric Imperative*, edited by A. R. Somers and D. R. Fabian. New York: Appleton-Century-Crofts, 1981.

Finch, R. H., and R. O. Egeberg. "A Report on the Health of the Nation's Health Care System." *National Archives and Records Service Weekly Compilation of Presidential Documents*, 5, No. 28 (14 July 1969), 963–969.

Fisher, C. "Differences by Age Groups in Health Care Spending." *Health Care Financing Review*, 1, No. 4 (Spring 1980), 65–90.

Frankel, B. "On the State of the State: Marxist Theories of the State After Leninism." In *Classes, Power and Conflict*, edited by A. Giddens and D. Held. Berkeley, Calif.: University of California Press, 1982.

Freeland, M. S., and C. E. Schendler. "National Health Expenditures: Short-Term Outlook and Long-Term Projections." *Health Care Financing Review*, 2, No. 3 (Winter 1981), 97–138.

Friedland, R., R. R. Alford, and F. F. Piven. "The Political Management of the Urban Fiscal Crisis." Paper presented at the annual meeting of the American Sociological Association, September, 1977, Chicago.

Friedman, M. *Capitalism and Freedom*. Chicago: University of Chicago Press, 1962.

Friedson, E. *Profession of Medicine*. New York: Dodd, Mead, 1970a.

_____. *Professional Dominance*. Chicago: Aldine, 1970b.

Fries, J. F. "Aging, Natural Death, and the Compression of Morbidity." *New England Journal of Medicine*, 303, No. 3 (17 July 1980), 130–135.

Fries, J. F., and L. M. Crapo. *Vitality and Aging*. San Francisco: Freeman, 1981.

Fuchs, V. R. "The Battle for Control of Health Care." *Health Affairs*, 1, No. 3 (Summer 1982), 5–13.

Garfield, J. "Social Stress and Medical Ideology." In *Stress and Survival*, edited by C. Garfield. St. Louis, Mo.: Mosby, 1979.

Gibson, R. M. "National Health Expenditures, 1979." *Health Care Financing Review*, 2, No. 1 (Summer 1980), 1–36.

Gibson, R. M., and D. R. Waldo. "National Health Expenditures, 1980." *Health Care Financing Review*, 3, No. 1 (September 1981), 1–54.

_____. "National Health Expenditures, 1981." *Health Care Financing Review*, 4, No. 1 (September 1982), 1–35.

Gibson, R. M., D. R. Waldo, and K. R. Levit. "National Health Expenditures, 1982." *Health Care Financing Review*, 5, No. 1 (Fall 1983), 1–31.

Giddens, A. *The Class Structure of the Advanced Societies*. New York: Harper and Row, 1975.

Giddens, A., and D. Held, eds. *Classes, Power and Conflict: Classical and Contemporary Debates*. Berkeley, Calif.: University of California Press, 1982.

Ginsberg, N. *Class, Capital and Social Policy*. London: Macmillan, 1979.

Ginzberg, E. "The Political Economy of Health." *Bulletin of the New York Academy of Medicine*, 41, No. 10 (October 1965), 1015–1036.

Gough, I. *The Political Economy of the Welfare State*. London: Macmillan, 1979.

Gouldner, A. *The Coming Crisis of Western Sociology*. New York: Basic, 1970.

Grad, S. *Income of the Population 55 and Over, 1980*. Washington, D.C.: U.S. Government Printing Office, 1983.

Grad, S., and K. Foster, "Income of the Population Aged 55 and Older, 1976." *Social Security Bulletin*, 42, No. 7 (July 1979), 16–32.

Graebner, W. *A History of Retirement*. New Haven, Conn.: Yale University Press, 1980.

Greenstein, R., and J. Bickerman. "The Effect of the Administration's Budget, Tax and Military Policies on Low Income Americans." Washington, D.C.: Interreligious Task Force on U.S. Food Policy, 1983.

Gruenberg, E. M. "The Failures of Success." *Milbank Memorial Fund Quarterly/ Health and Society*, 55, No. 1 (1977), 3–24.

Gubrium, J. F. *The Myth of the Golden Years: A Socio-Environmental Theory of Aging*. Springfield, Ill.: Charles C. Thomas, 1973.

Guillemard, A. M. "Retirement as a Social Process: Its Differential Effects Upon Behavior." Communication presented to the Eighth World Congress of Sociology, August 21, 1974, Toronto.

_____. "Old Age, Retirement, and the Social Class Structure: Toward an Analysis of the Structural Dynamics of the Latter Stage of Life." In *Aging and Life Course Transitions: An Interdisciplinary Perspective*, edited by T. K. Hareven and K. J. Adams. New York: Guildford, 1982.

_____. "The Making of Old Age Policy in France." In *Old Age and the Welfare State*, edited by A. M. Guillemard. New York: International Sociological Association, 1983.

Gusfield, J. R. *Symbolic Crusade*. Champagne, Ill.: University of Illinois Press, 1966.

_____. "Categories of Ownership and Responsibility in Social Issues: Alcohol Abuse and Automobile Use." *Journal of Drug Issues*, 5 (Fall 1975), 285–303.

Haber, C. *Beyond Sixty-Five: The Dilemma of Old Age in America's Past*. London: Cambridge University Press, 1983.

Hadley, J. *More Medical Care, Better Health?* Washington, D.C.: Urban Institute, 1982.

Harrington, C. "Public Policy Issues: The Nursing Home Industry," AHPC Working Paper No. 16. San Francisco: Aging Health Policy Center, University of California, 1982.

_____. "Social Security and Medicare: Policy Shifts in the 1980s." In *Fiscal Austerity and Aging*, by C. L. Estes, R. J. Newcomer, et al. Beverly Hills, Calif.: Sage, 1983.

Harris, L. *The Myth and Reality of Aging in America*. Washington, D.C.: National Council on the Aging, 1975.

Harris, R. *A Sacred Trust*. Baltimore: Penguin, 1969.

Havemann, J. "Sharing the Wealth: The Gap Between Rich and Poor Grows Wider." *National Journal*, 14, No. 43 (23 October 1982), 1788–1795.

Havighurst, R. J., and R. Albrecht. *Older People*. New York: Longmans B. Green, 1953.

Havighurst, R. J., J. M. A. Munnichs, B. Neugarten, and H. Thomae. *Adjustment to Retirement*. Assen, The Netherlands: Van Gorcum, 1969.

Hendricks, J., and C. D. Hendricks. *Aging in Mass Society: Myths and Realities*. Cambridge, Mass.: Winthrop, 1981.

Henretta, J., and R. Campbell. "Status Attainment and Status Maintenance: A Case Study of Stratification in Old Age." *American Sociological Review*, 41 (1976), 981–992.

Hess, B., and E. Markson. *Aging and Old Age*. New York: Macmillan, 1980.

Hickey, T. *Health and Aging*. Monterey, Calif.: Brooks/Cole, 1980.

Hiestand, D. L. "Pluralism in Health Services." In *Urban Health Services*, edited by E. Ginzberg. New York: Columbia University Press, 1971.

Hodgson, G. "The Politics of American Health Care." *The Atlantic Monthly*, 232, No. 4 (October 1973), 45–61.

Holahan, J. *Financing Health Care for the Poor*. Lexington, Mass.: Heath, 1975.

Holahan, J., W. Scanlon, and B. Spitz. "Public Finance: Impact of National Economic Conditions on Health Care of the Poor." Washington, D.C.: Urban Institute, 1980.

Holtzman, A. *The Townsend Movement*. New York: Bookman, 1963.

Hoos, I. R. *Systems Analysis in Public Policy: A Critique*. Berkeley, Calif.: University of California Press, 1972.

Hunter, F. *Community Power Structure*. Chapel Hill, N.C.: University of North Carolina Press, 1953.

Iglehart, J. K. "Health Care and American Business." *The New England Journal of Medicine*, 306, No. 2 (14 January 1982), 120–124.

Jackson, K. T., and S. K. Schultz, eds. *Cities in American History*. New York: Knopf, 1972.

John, R. "What is an Adequate Theory of Aging?" Paper presented at the meeting of the International Sociological Association, 1982, Mexico City.

Kane, R. A., and R. L. Kane. *Assessing the Elderly: A Practical Guide to Measurement*. Lexington, Mass.: Heath, 1981.

_____. "Long-Term Care: A Field in Search of Values." In *Values and Long Term Care*, edited by R. L. Kane and R. A. Kane. Lexington, Mass.: Heath, 1982.

Kart, C. S., and B. L. Beckham. "Black-White Differentials in the Institutionalization of the Elderly: A Temporal Analysis." *Social Forces*, 54, No. 4 (1976), 901–910.

Kasper, J. A. "Prescribed Medicines: Use, Expenditures, and Sources of Payment." In *Data Preview 9, National Health Care Expenditure Study*. Washington, D.C.: U.S. National Center for Health Services Research, DHHS, 1982.

Kelman, S. "Toward the Political Economy of Medical Care." *Inquiry*, 8, No. 3 (September 1971), 30–38.

Kelman, S., ed. "Special Section on Political Economy of Health." *International Journal of Health Services*, 5, No. 4 (1975), 535–642.

Keynes, J. M. *General Theory of Employment, Interest & Money*. New York: Harcourt, 1965.

Kissick, W. L. "Health Manpower in Transition." In *Economic Aspects of Health Care*, edited by J. B. McKinlay. New York: Prodist, 1973.

Kitagawa, E. M., and P. M. Hauser. *Differential Mortality in the United States*. Cambridge, Mass.: Harvard University Press, 1973.

Kleinman, J. C., M. Gold, and D. Makuc. "Use of Ambulatory Medical Care by the Poor: Another Look at Equity." *Medical Care*, 19, No. 10 (October 1981), 1011–1029.

Klemmack, D. L., and L. L. Roff. "Predicting General Comparative Support for Government's Providing Benefits to Older Persons." *Gerontologist*, 21, No. 6 (December 1981), 592–599.

Koff, T. H. *Long-Term Care: An Approach to Serving the Frail Elderly.* Boston: Little, Brown, 1982.

Kramer, M. "The Rising Pandemic of Mental Disorders and Associated Chronic Diseases and Disabilities." *Acta Psychiatrica Scandinavica*, 62, Suppl. 285 (1980), 382–397.

Kreps, J., and R. Clark. *Sex, Age, and Work.* Baltimore: Johns Hopkins, 1975.

Kuypers, J. A., and V. L. Bengston. "Social Breakdown and Competence: A Model of Normal Aging." *Human Development*, 16, No. 3 (1973), 181–201.

Langer, E. J. "Old Age: An Artifact?" In *Aging: Biology and Behavior*, edited by J. L. McGaugh and S. B. Kiesler. New York: Academic, 1981.

Langer, E. J., and J. Rodin. "The Effects of Choice and Enhanced Personal Responsibility for the Aged." *Journal of Personality and Social Psychology*, 34 (1976), 191–198.

Law, S. *Blue Cross: What Went Wrong?* New Haven, Conn.: Yale University Press, 1974.

Leadership Council of Aging Organizations. *The Administration's 1984 Budget: A Critical View from an Aging Perspective.* Washington, D.C.: LCAO, March 1983.

Lee, P. R. "A New Perspective on Health, Health Planning, and Health Policy." *Journal of Allied Health*, 6, No. 1 (Winter 1977), 8–15.

———. "Fiscal Crisis in Medicine." Grand rounds presented to the Department of Dermatology, School of Medicine, University of California, San Francisco, March 30, 1983.

Lee, P. R., and H. L. Lipton. *Drugs and the Elderly: A Background Paper*, Policy Paper No. 3. San Francisco: Aging Health Policy Center and Institute for Health Policy Studies, University of California, 1982.

Lehrman, R. "Poverty Statistics Serve as Nagging Reminder." *Generations: Journal of the Western Gerontological Society*, 4, No. 1 (May 1980), 17.

LeRoy, L. "The Political Economy of U.S. Federal Health Policy: A Closer Look at Medicare." Unpublished manuscript, Health Policy Institute, University of California, San Francisco, 1979.

Little, V. *Open Care for the Aging.* New York: Springer, 1982.

Liu, K., and J. Mossey. "The Role of Payment Source in Differentiating Nursing Home Residents, Services, and Payments." *Health Care Financing Review*, 2, No. 1 (Summer 1980), 51–61.

Long, S. H., R. F. Settle, and C. R. Link. "Who Bears the Burden of Medicare Cost Sharing?" *Inquiry*, 19 (Fall 1982), 222–234.

Lowenthal, M. F. "Psychosocial Variations Across the Adult Life Course: Frontiers for Research and Policy." *Gerontologist*, 15, No. 1, Pt. 1 (February 1975), 6–12.

Lowi, T. *The End of Liberalism.* New York: Norton, 1969.

————. *The Politics of Disorder*. New York: Basic, 1971.

Lubove, R. *The Struggle for Social Security: 1900–1935*. Cambridge, Mass.: Harvard University Press, 1968.

Luft, H. S. *Poverty and Health: Economic Causes and Consequences of Health Problems*. Cambridge, Mass.: Ballinger, 1978.

————. *Health Maintenance Organizations: Dimensions of Performance*. New York: Wiley, 1981.

Magaziner, I., and R. Reich. *Minding America's Business: The Decline and Rise of the American Economy*. New York: Harcourt Brace Jovanovich, 1982.

Mandel, E. *The Second Slump: A Marxist Analysis of Recession in the Seventies*. London: NLB, 1978.

Manton, K. G. "Changing Concepts of Morbidity and Mortality in the Elderly Population." *Health and Society*, 60, No. 2 (1982), 183–244.

Markson, E. W., and J. Hand. "Referral for Death: Low Status of the Aged and Referral for Psychiatric Hospitalization." *Aging and Human Development*, 1 (1970), 261–272.

Marmor, T. *The Politics of Medicare*. New Haven, Conn.: Yale University Press, 1970.

Marshall, T. H. *Class, Citizenship, and Social Development*. New York: Doubleday, 1964.

Marshall, V. W., ed. *Aging in Canada: Social Perspectives*. Ontario: Fitzhenry and Whiteside, 1980.

Massachusetts Institute of Technology (M.I.T.). *Work in America*. Cambridge, Mass.: M.I.T. Press, 1973.

Matza, D. *Becoming Deviant*. Englewood Cliffs, N.J.: Prentice Hall, 1969.

McAdam, D. "Coping with Aging or Combatting Agism?" In *Aging: Coping with Medical Issues*, edited by A. Kolker and P. Ahmed. New York: Elsevier, 1982.

McGaugh, J. L., and S. B. Kiesler. *Aging: Biology and Behavior*. New York: Academic, 1981.

McIntyre, R. S., and D. C. Tipps. *Inequity and Decline*. Washington, D.C.: Center on Budget and Policy Priorities, 1983.

McKenzie, S. *Aging and Old Age*. Glenview, Ill.: Scott, Foresman, 1980.

McKeown, T. "Determinants of Health." *Human Nature*, 1, No. 4 (April 1978), 60–67.

McKinlay, J. B. "A Case for Refocusing Upstream: The Political Economy of Illness." In *The Sociology of Health and Illness—Critical Perspectives*, edited by P. Conrad and R. Kern. New York: St. Martin's, 1981.

McKinlay, J. B., and S. M. McKinlay. "The Questionable Contribution of Medical Measures to the Decline of Mortality in the United States in the Twentieth Century." *Milbank Memorial Fund Quarterly/Health and Society*, 55 (Summer 1977), 405–428.

————. "Medical Measures and the Decline of Mortality." In *The Sociology of Health and Illness—Critical Perspectives*, edited by P. Conrad and R. Kern. New York: St. Martin's, 1981.

Miller, S. M. "The Political Economy of Social Problems: From the Sixties to the Seventies." *Social Problems*, 23, No. 1 (1976), 131–141.

Mills, C. W. *The Power Elite*. New York: Oxford University Press, 1956.

Minkler, M. "Blaming the Aged Victim: The Politics of Scapegoating in Times of Fiscal Conservatism." *International Journal of Health Services*, 13, No. 1 (1983), 155–168.

Morison, S. E., and H. S. Commager. *The Growth of the American Republic*, Vol. 2. New York: Oxford University Press, 1962.

Munnichs, J. M. A., and W. J. A. van den Huevel, eds. *Dependency or Interdependency in Old Age*. The Hague: Martinus Nijhoff, 1976.

Munts, R. *Bargaining for Health*. Madison, Wis.: University of Wisconsin Press, 1967.

Myles, J. F. "The Aged, the State, and the Structure of Inequality." In *Structural Inequality in Canada*, edited by J. Harp and J. Hofley. Toronto: Prentice–Hall, 1980.

_____. "The Aged and the Welfare State: An Essay in Political Demography." Paper presented at the International Sociological Association, July 8–9, 1981, Paris.

_____. "Population Aging and the Elderly." In *Social Issues: Sociological Views of Canada*, edited by D. Forcese and S. Richer. Ontario: Prentice-Hall, 1982.

_____. *The Political Economy of Public Pensions*. Boston: Little, Brown, 1984.

Najman, J. M. "Theories of Disease Causation and the Concept of a General Susceptibility: A Review." *Social Science and Medicine*, 14A, No. 3 (May 1980), 231–237.

Navarro, V. "Health and the Corporate Society." *Social Policy*, 5, No. 5 (January/February 1975a), 41–49.

_____. "The Political Economy of Medical Care." *International Journal of Health Services*, 5, No. 1 (1975b), 65–94.

_____. *Medicine Under Capitalism*. New York: Prodist, 1976.

_____. *Health and Medical Care in the U.S.: A Critical Analysis*. New York: Baywood, 1977.

Nelson, G. "Social Class and Public Policy for the Elderly." *Social Service Review*, 56, No. 1 (March 1982), 85–107.

_____. "Tax Expenditures for the Elderly." *Gerontologist*, 23, No. 5 (October 1983), 471–478.

Neugarten, B. L., R. J. Havighurst, and S. S. Tobin. "Personality and Patterns of Aging." In *Middle Age and Aging*, edited by B. L. Neugarten. Chicago: University of Chicago Press, 1968.

Neugarten, B. L., et al., eds. *Personality in Middle and Late Life*. New York: Atherton, 1964.

New York State Office on Aging. *Medicine: Analysis and Recommendations for Reform*. Albany, N.Y.: N.Y. State Office on Aging, September 1983.

Newcomer, R. J., and C. Harrington. "State Medicaid Expenditures: Trends and Program Policy Changes." In *Fiscal Austerity and Aging*, by C. L. Estes, R. J. Newcomer, et al. Beverly Hills, Calif.: Sage, 1983.

O'Connor, J. *The Fiscal Crisis of the State*. New York: St. Martin's, 1973.

Offe, C., and V. Ronge. "Thesis on the Theory of the State." In *Classes, Power and Conflict*, edited by A. Giddens and D. Held. Berkeley, Calif.: University of California Press, 1982.

Olson, L. K. *The Political Economy of Aging*. New York: Columbia University Press, 1982.

Olson, L., C. Caton, and M. Duffy. *The Elderly and the Future Economy*. Lexington, Mass.: Lexington/Heath, 1981.

Palmer, J., and I. Sawhill, eds. *The Reagan Experiment*. Washington, D.C.: Urban Institute, 1982.

Parsons, T. *The Social System*. New York: Free Press, 1951.

Piven, F. F., and R. Cloward. *The New Class War*. New York: Pantheon, 1982.

Powles, J. "On the Limitations of Modern Medicine." *Science, Medicine, and Man*, 1, No. 1 (1973), 1–30.

Pratt, H. J. *The Gray Lobby*. Chicago: University of Chicago Press, 1976.

Prentice, R. "Patterns of Psychoactive Drug Use Among the Elderly." In *The Aging Process and Psychoactive Drug Use*. Washington, D.C.: U.S. Government Printing Office, 1979.

Ragan, P. K., and W. J. Davis. "The Diversity of Older Voters." *Society*, 15, No. 5 (July/August 1978), 50–53.

Ragan, P. K., and J. B. Wales. "Age Stratification and the Life Course." In *Handbook of Mental Health and Aging*, edited by J. E. Birren and R. B. Sloane. Englewood Cliffs, N.J.: Prentice-Hall, 1980.

Rahn, R. W., and K. D. Simonson. "Tax Policy for Retirement Programs." In *Retirement Income: Who Gets How Much and Who Pays?* (National Journal Issues Book). Washington, D.C.: Government Research Corporation, 1980.

Rawls, J. *Theory of Justice*. Cambridge, Mass.: Belknap/Harvard Press, 1971.

Relman, A. S. "The New Medical-Industrial Complex." *New England Journal of Medicine*, 303, No. 17 (23 October 1980), 963–970.

Renaud, M. "On the Structural Constraints to State Intervention in Health." *International Journal of Health Services*, 5, No. 4 (1975), 559–571.

Ricardo-Campbell, R. *The Economics and Politics of Health*. Chapel Hill, N.C.: University of North Carolina, 1982.

Rice, D. P., and J. J. Feldman. "Living Longer in the United States: Demographic Changes and Health Needs of the Elderly." *Milbank Memorial Fund Quarterly/Health and Society*, 61, No. 3 (1983), 362–396.

Riley, M. W., M. Johnson, and A. Foner. "A Sociology of Age Stratification." In *Aging and Society*, Vol. 3, edited by M. W. Riley et al. New York: Basic, 1972.

Rimlinger, G. V. *Welfare Policy and Industrialization in Europe, America, and Russia*. New York: John Wiley, 1971.

Rodberg, L. and G. Stevenson. "The Health Care Industry in Advanced Capitalism." *The Review of Radical Political Economics*, 9, No. 1 (Spring 1977), 104–115.

Rodin, J., and E. Langer. "Long-Term Effects of a Control-Relevant Intervention with the Institutionalized Aged." *Journal of Personality and Social Psychology*, 35 (1977), 897–902.

_____. "Aging Labels: The Decline of Control and the Fall of Self-Esteem." *The Journal of Social Issues*, 36, No. 2 (Spring 1980), 12–29.

Roosevelt, F. D. *Public Papers and Addresses*, Vol. 3. New York: Random House, 1938.

Rose, A. M. *The Power Structure: Political Process in American Society*. London: Oxford University Press, 1967.

Rosenblum, M. "The Last Push: From Discouraged Work to Inventory Retirement." *Industrial Gerontology*, 1, No. 1 (Winter 1975), 14–22.

Ross, D., and W. Birdsall. *Social Security and Pensions* (U.S. Special Study on Economic Change). Washington, D.C.: U.S. Congress, Joint Economic Committee, 1980.

Rudov, M. H., and N. Santangelo. *Health Status of Minorities and Low-Income Groups*. Washington, D.C.: U.S. Government Printing Office, 1979.

Ruther, M., and A. Dobson. "Equal Treatment and Unequal Benefits: A Re-Examination of the Use of Medicare Services by Race, 1967–1976." *Health Care Financing Review*, 2, No. 3 (Winter 1981), 55–83.

Ryan, W. *Blaming the Victim*. New York: Vintage, 1971.

_____. *Equality*. New York: Vintage, 1982.

Salmon, J. W. "Monopoly Capital and the Reorganization of the Health Sector." *The Review of Radical Political Economics*, 9, No. 1 (Spring 1977), 125–133.

_____. "The Competitive Health Strategy: Fighting for Your Health." *Health and Medicine*, 1, No. 2 (Spring 1982), 21–30.

Samuelson, R. J. "Busting the U.S. Budget: The Costs of an Aging America." *National Journal*, 10, No. 7 (18 February 1978), 256–260.

_____. "Benefit Programs for the Elderly Off Limits to Federal Budget Cutters?" *National Journal*, 13, No. 40 (3 October 1981), 1757–1762.

Schur, E. *Labeling Deviant Behavior*. New York: Harper and Row, 1971.

Scitovsky, A. "Equity of Access to Health Care." Paper presented at the University of California, San Francisco, November, 1982.

Sclar, E. "Aging and Economic Development." In *Public Policies for an Aging Population*, edited by E. W. Markson and G. R. Batra. Lexington, Mass.: Heath, 1980.

Scott, R. *The Making of Blind Men*. New York: Russell Sage Foundation, 1970.

Scull, A. T. *Decarceration*. Englewood Cliffs, N.J.: Prentice-Hall, 1977.

Sjoberg, G., R. A. Brymer, and B. Farris. "Bureaucracy and the Lower Class." *Sociology and Social Research*, 50 (1966), 325–334.

Skocpol, T., and J. Ikenberry. "The Political Formation of the American Welfare State in Historical and Comparative Perspective." Paper presented at the annual meeting of the American Sociological Association, September 7, 1982, San Francisco.

Somers, A. R., and D. R. Fabian. *The Geriatric Imperative*. New York: Appleton-Century-Crofts, 1981.

Spector, M., and J. Kitsuse. *Constructing Social Problems*. Menlo Park, Calif.: Benjamin-Cummings, 1979.

Spiegel, A. D., and S. Podair, eds. *Medicaid: Lessons for National Health Insurance*. Rockville, Md.: Aspen, 1975.

Stacey, M., and H. Homans. "Sociology of Health and Illness: Its Present State, Future Prospects and Potential for Health Research." *Sociology*, 12, No. 2 (September 1978), 281–307.

Starr, P. *The Social Transformation of American Medicine*. New York: Basic, 1982.

Stephens, R. C., C. A. Haney, and S. Underwood. "Psychoactive Drug Use and Potential Misuse Among Persons Aged 55 Years and Older." In *Drugs,*

Alcohol and Aging, edited by D. M. Petersen and F. J. Whittington. Dubuque, Iowa: Kendall/Hunt, 1982, 75–83.

Stevens, S., and R. Stevens. *Welfare Medicine in America*. New York: Free Press/ Macmillan, 1974.

Stewart, W. H. "Health Services: Who's in Charge?" The HEW Forum Papers: 1967–1968. Washington, D.C.: U.S. Government Printing Office, 1968.

Storey, J. R. *Older Americans in the Reagan Era: Impacts of Federal Policy Changes*. Washington, D.C.: Urban Institute, 1983.

Strauss, R. "The Nature and Status of Medical Sociology." *American Sociological Review*, 22, No. 2 (1957), 200–204.

Syme, S. L., and L. F. Berkman. "Social Class, Susceptibility, and Sickness." *American Journal of Epidemiology*, 104 (July 1976), 1–8.

Thomas, W. I. *The Unadjusted Girl*. Santa Fe, N. Mex.: Gannor, 1970.

Thurow, L. *The Zero Sum Society*. New York: Penguin, 1981.

Titmuss, R. "The Role of Redistribution in Social Policy." *Social Security Bulletin*, 28 (June 1965), 14–20.

Tobin, J. "Reaganomics and Economics." *New York Review of Books*, 28, No. 19 (3 December 1981), 11–14.

Torrens, P. R. "Historical Evolution and Overview of Health Services in the United States." In *Introduction to Health Services*, edited by S. J. Williams and P. R. Torrens. New York: Wiley, 1980.

Townsend, P. *Poverty in the United Kingdom*. Berkeley, Calif.: University of California Press, 1979.

———. "The Structured Dependency of the Elderly: A Creation of Social Policy in the Twentieth Century." *Ageing and Society*, 1, No. 1 (1981), 5–28.

Tussing, A. "The Dual Welfare System." In *Social Realities*, edited by L. Horowitz and C. Levey. New York: Harper and Row, 1971.

Twaddle, A. "From Medical Sociology to the Sociology of Health." In *Sociology: The State of the Art*, edited by T. Bottomore, S. Nowak, and M. Sokdowska. Beverly Hills, Calif.: Sage, 1982.

U.S. Bureau of the Census. *Money Income and Poverty Status of Families and Persons in the United States: 1980*. Washington, D.C.: U.S. Government Printing Office, 1981.

———. *Money Income and Poverty Status of Families and Persons in the United States: 1981*. Washington, D.C.: U.S. Government Printing Office, 1982.

———. *Statistical Abstract of the United States: 1982–1983*. Washington, D.C.: U.S. Government Printing Office, 1983.

U.S. Congressional Budget Office (CBO). *Economic Policy and the Outlook for the Economy*. Washington, D.C.: U.S. CBO, 1981a.

———. *Medicaid: Choices for 1982 and Beyond*. Washington, D.C.: U.S. CBO, 1981b.

———. *Effects of Tax and Benefit Reductions Enacted in 1981 for Households in Different Income Categories*. Washington, D.C.: U.S. CBO, 1982a.

———. *Effects of Tax and Benefit Payments Enacted in 1982 for Households in Different Income Categories*. Washington, D.C.: U.S. CBO, 1982b.

———. *Tax Expenditures: Budget Control Options and Five-Year Budget Projections for FY 1983–1987*. Washington, D.C.: U.S. CBO, 1982c.

_____. *Changing the Structure of Medicare Benefits: Issues and Options*. Washington, D.C.: U.S. CBO, 1983.

U.S. Congress, Joint Committee on Taxation. *Estimates of Federal Tax Expenditures for Fiscal Years 1983–1988*. Washington, D.C.: U.S. Government Printing Office, March 1983.

U.S. Department of Health, Education, and Welfare (DHEW). *Towards a Comprehensive Health Policy for the 1970's*. Washington, D.C.: U.S. Government Printing Office, 1971.

_____. *Forward Plan for Health: FY 1978–1982*. Washington, D.C.: U.S. Government Printing Office, 1976.

_____. *Income and Resources of the Aged*. Washington, D.C.: U.S. Government Printing Office, 1980.

U.S. General Accounting Office (GAO). *Home Health—The Need for a National Policy to Better Provide for the Elderly*. Washington, D.C.: U.S. GAO, 1977.

_____. *Entering a Nursing Home—Costly Implications for Medicaid and the Elderly*. Report to the Congress by the Comptroller General of the United States. Washington, D.C.: U.S. GAO, 1979.

_____. *Perspective on Income Security and Social Services and an Agenda for Analysis*. Washington, D.C.: U.S. GAO, August 1981.

_____. *A Primer on Competitive Strategies for Containing Health Care Costs*. Washington, D.C.: U.S. GAO, September 1982.

U.S. House, Committee on the Budget. *President Reagan's Fiscal Year 1984 Budget*. Washington, D.C.: U.S. Government Printing Office, February 1983.

U.S. House, Committee on Government Operations. *Current Condition of American Federalism*. Washington, D.C.: U.S. Government Printing Office, 1981.

U.S. House, Committee on Post Office and Civil Service. Subcommittee on Census and Population. *Impact of Budget Cuts on Federal Statistical Programs*. Washington, D.C.: U.S. Government Printing Office, March 1982.

U.S. House, Committee on Ways and Means. *Elimination of Minimum Social Security Benefit Under Public Law*. Washington, D.C.: U.S. Government Printing Office, 1981.

_____. *National Health Care Expenditures and Expenditures for Health Care by the Elderly*. Washington, D.C.: U.S. Government Printing Office, 1982.

U.S. House, Select Committee on Aging. *Poverty Among America's Aged*. Washington, D.C.: U.S. Government Printing Office, August 1978.

_____. *Analysis of the Impact of the Proposed Fiscal Year 1982 Budget Cuts on the Elderly*. Washington, D.C.: U.S. Government Printing Office, 1981.

_____. *The Unemployment Crisis Facing Older Americans*. Washington, D.C.: U.S. Government Printing Office, October 1982.

U.S. National Institute on Aging (NIA). *The Older Woman: Continuities and Discontinuities*. Washington, D.C.: U.S. Department of Health, Education and Welfare, National Institutes of Health, October 1979.

U.S. President's Commission for the Study of Ethical Problems in Medicine and Biomedical and Behavioral Research. *Securing Access to Health Care: A Report on the Ethical Implications of Differences in the Availability of Health*

Services, Vol. 1. Washington, D.C.: U.S. Government Printing Office, 1983.

U.S. Public Law 96-499. *The Omnibus Reconciliation Act of 1980*. Washington, D.C.: U.S. Government Printing Office, 1980.

U.S. Public Law 97-35. *The Omnibus Budget Reconciliation Act of 1981*. Washington, D.C.: U.S. Government Printing Office, 1981.

U.S. Senate, Committee on Finance. *Health Benefits: Loss Due to Unemployment*. Washington, D.C.: U.S. Government Printing Office, April 1983.

U.S. Senate, Committee on Veterans' Affairs. *Study of Health Care for American Veterans*. Washington, D.C.: U.S. Government Printing Office, 7 June 1977a.

_____. *Veterans Administration's Response to the Study of Health Care for American Veterans*. Washington, D.C.: U.S. Government Printing Office, 22 September 1977b.

U.S. Senate, Special Committee on Aging. *Nursing Home Care in the U.S.: Failure in Public Policy* (Introductory Report and Supporting Papers, Nos. 1–7). Washington, D.C.: U.S. Government Printing Office, 1974–1976.

_____. *Developments in Aging: 1979* (Senate Report No. 96-613). Washington, D.C.: U.S. Government Printing Office, 1980.

_____. *Developments in Aging: 1980* (Senate Report No. 97-62). Washington, D.C.: U.S. Government Printing Office, 1981.

_____. *Developments in Aging: 1981* (Senate Report No. 97-314). Washington, D.C.: U.S. Government Printing Office, 1982a.

_____. *The Proposed Fiscal Year 1983 Budget: What It Means for Older Americans*. Washington, D.C.: U.S. Government Printing Office, 1982b.

_____. *The Future of Medicare*. Washington, D.C.: U.S. Government Printing Office, 1983a.

_____. *The Proposed Fiscal Year 1984 Budget: What It Means for Older Americans*. Washington, D.C.: U.S. Government Printing Office, 1983b.

_____. *Developments in Aging: 1982* (Senate Report No. 98-13, Vol. 1). Washington, D.C.: U.S. Government Printing Office, 1983c.

Urquhart, M. "The Service Industry: Is it Recession Proof?" *Monthly Labor Review*, 104 (1981), 12–18.

Vladeck, B. C. *Unloving Care: The Nursing Home Tragedy*. New York: Basic, 1980.

_____. "Equity, Access, and the Costs of Health Services." *Medical Care*, 19, No. 12, Suppl. (December 1981a), 69–80.

_____. "The Market vs. Regulation: The Case for Regulation." *Milbank Memorial Fund Quarterly/Health and Society*, 59, No. 2 (1981b), 209–223.

Waitzkin, H. "The Marxist Paradigm in Medicine." *International Journal of Health Services*, 9, No. 4 (1979), 683–698.

_____. *The Second Sickness: Contradictions of Capitalist Health Care*. New York: Free Press/Macmillan, 1983.

Waitzkin, H., and B. Waterman. *The Exploitation of Illness in Capitalist Society*. New York: Bobbs-Merrill, 1974.

Walker, A. "The Social Creation of Poverty and Dependency in Old Age." *Journal of Social Policy*, 9, No. 1 (1980), 49–75.

_____. "Towards a Political Economy of Old Age." *Ageing and Society*, 1, No. 1 (1981), 73–94.

Walker, D. *Toward a Functioning Federalism*. Cambridge, Mass.: Winthrop, 1981.

Wallace, D. J. "The Biology of Aging: 1976, An Overview." *Journal of the American Geriatrics Society*, 25, No. 3 (1977), 104–111.

Walton, J. "Urban Political Economy." *Comparative Urban Research*, 7, No. 1 (1979), 5–17.

Weber, M. "Class, Status and Party." In *From Max Weber: Essays in Sociology*, edited and translated by H. H. Gerth and C. W. Mills. New York: Oxford University Press, 1946.

Weinstein, J. *The Corporate Ideal in the Liberal State: 1900–1918*. Boston: Beacon, 1968.

Whitt, J. A. "Toward a Class-Dialectical Model of Power: An Empirical Assessment of Three Competing Models of Political Power." *American Sociological Review*, 44 (February 1979), 81–100.

Wilensky, G. R. "Government and the Financing of Health Care." *Government and Health*, 72, No. 2 (May 1982), 202–207.

Williamson, J. "Public Policy and Regulation of the Elderly Poor Prior to the Rise of the Welfare State." Paper presented to the Society for the Study of Social Problems, September, 1982, San Francisco.

Wright, E. O. *Class, Crisis and the State*. London: Verso, 1978.

Zola, I. K. "In the Name of Health and Illness: On Some Socio-Political Consequences of Medical Influence." *Social Science and Medicine*, 9, No. 2 (February 1975), 83–87.

_____. *Disabling Professions*. Boston: Marion Boyers, 1977.

Author Index

Najman, J. M., 84
Navarro, V., 14, 15, 23, 24, 112
Nelson, G., 2, 52, 96, 100, 104
Neugarten, B. L., 8
New York State Office on Aging, 108
Newcomer, R. J., 89, 109

O'Connor, J., 24, 28, 65
Offe, C., 24
Olson, L., 74
Olson, L. K., 2, 16

Palmer, J., 104
Parsons, T., 5, 21
Piven, F. F., 112
Powles, J., 18
Pratt, H. J., 44, 45
Prentice, R., 89

Ragan, P. K., 9
Rahn, R. W., 26
Relman, A. S., 19, 66, 95
Renaud, M., 15, 18
Ricardo-Campbell, R., 56, 67
Rice, D. P., 76, 81
Riley, M. W., 9
Rimlinger, G. V., 40, 42, 43, 44, 48, 49
Rodberg, L., 62
Rodin, J., 4, 5
Roosevelt, F. D., 45
Rose, A. M., 48, 49
Rosenblum, M., 73
Ross, D., 74
Rudov, M. H., 79
Ruther, M., 84

Salmon, J. W., 69, 70, 98
Schur, E., 4
Sclar, E., 90
Scott, R., 4

Scull, A. T., 19, 65
Sjoberg, G., 33
Skocpol, T., 37, 38, 42, 46
Somers, A. R., 10
Stacey, M., 15
Starr, P., 40, 43, 44, 47, 48, 65, 67, 69, 111, 112, 114
Stephens, R. C., 89
Stevens, S., 46, 50–52
Stewart, W. H., 60, 61
Storey, J. R., 73, 75, 105, 106
Strauss, R., 15
Syme, S. L., 84

Thomas, W. I., 4
Thurow, L., 105
Titmuss, R., 96
Tobin, J., 45
Townsend, P., 2, 16, 31, 75, 87
Tussing, A., 100
Twaddle, A., 15, 16

U.S. President's Commission, 115
Urquhart, M., 74

Vladeck, B. C., 68, 88, 89, 90, 99

Waitzkin, H., 16
Walker, A., 2, 12, 16, 31, 71–73, 100
Walker, D., 38, 46
Wallace, D. J., 7
Walton, J., 1
Weber, M., 2, 22, 24
Weinstein, J., 40
Whitt, J. A., 23
Wilensky, G. R., 52, 104
Williamson, J., 37, 38, 87
Wright, E. O., 30, 32

Zola, I. K., 5, 17

Subject Index